Clinical Focus on
Male and Female Infertility

Dedicated to

*Our parents, teachers, and all practicing
Obstetricians and Gynecologists*

Contributors

Anu Agarwal MD (Obs & Gyne) FIAMS
Director
Vansh Fertility and
Test Tube Baby Centre
Ayushman Multispecialty Hospital
Varanasi, Uttar Pradesh, India

Deeba Khanam MS
Assistant Professor
Department of Obstetrics and Gynecology
Aligarh Muslim University
Aligarh, Uttar Pradesh, India

Divya Yadav MD
Associate Professor
Department of Obstetrics and Gynecology
Sarojini Naidu Medical College
Agra, Uttar Pradesh, India

Jaideep Malhotra MD FICMCH FICOG FRCOG FRCPI FMAS
Managing Director
ART Rainbow IVF and MNMH (P) Ltd and
Ujala Cygnus Rainbow Hospital
Agra, Uttar Pradesh, India
President, SAFOM/ISPAT
Past President, IMS/ISAR/FOGSI/ASPIRE

Jaya Sharma MD
Director
Noble IVF and Rajmata Hospital
Aligarh, Uttar Pradesh, India

Keshav Malhotra MBBS MCE
Senior Consultant ESHRE Certified
Managing Director, ART Rainbow IVF
Managing Director, META
Director, Ujala Cygnus Rainbow Hospital
Director, MNMH (P) Ltd
Agra, Uttar Pradesh, India

Maneesha Jain MBBS MS FICOG FICMCH
Consultant
Galaxy IVF and Maternity Centre
Moradabad, Uttar Pradesh, India

Narendra Malhotra MD FICMCH FICOG FRCOG FICS FMAS FIAP
Managing Director
Global Rainbow Health Care and MNMH (P) Ltd
and Ujala Cygnus Rainbow Hospital
Agra, Uttar Pradesh, India
Professor, Sarajevo School of Science and Technology, Croatia
Past President, FOGSI/IFUMB/ISPAT/ISAR, INSARG
Vice President, WAPM/SAFOG
Director, International IAN Donald School and SAFOG

Neharika Malhotra MD (Gold Medalist) DRM (Germany) FICMCH Fellow ICOG (Rep Med) ICOG (USG)
Director and Consultant
ART Rainbow IVF and MNMH (P) Ltd and
Ujala Cygnus Rainbow Hospital
Agra, Uttar Pradesh, India
Joint Secretary, FOGSI
Chair, YTP Committee, FOGSI

Rehana Najam DGO MS Fellowship in ART FICOG
Professor and Head
Department of Obstetrics and Gynecology
Teerthanker Mahaveer Medical College
and Research Centre
Moradabad, Uttar Pradesh, India

Rekha Rani MD
Professor
Department of Obstetrics and Gynecology
Sarojini Naidu Medical College
Agra, Uttar Pradesh, India

Ruchika Garg MD
Professor
Department of Obstetrics and Gynecology
Sarojini Naidu Medical College
Agra, Uttar Pradesh, India
Joint Editor, Journal of SAFOG

Saeeda Wasim MBBS MS
FNB (Reproductive Medicine)
Head Consultant
Nova IVF Fertility Center
Lucknow, Uttar Pradesh, India

Shaheen Anjum MS ACME (Advance Course in Medical Education) Fellowship in Reproductive Medicine
Professor and In-charge ART Unit
Department of Obstetrics and Gynecology
JN Medical College, Aligarh Muslim University
Aligarh, Uttar Pradesh, India

Sharique Ahmad MD
Professor
Department of Pathology
Era's Lucknow Medical College and Hospital
Era University
Lucknow, Uttar Pradesh, India

Shikha Sachan MD (Obs & Gyne)
Associate Professor
Department of Obstetrics and Gynecology
Institute of Medical Sciences
Banaras Hindu University
Varanasi, Uttar Pradesh, India

Shikha Seth MD FICS FICOG
Professor and Head
Department of Obstetrics and Gynecology
All India Institute of Medical Sciences
Gorakhpur, Uttar Pradesh, India

Sufia Naseem MD
Assistant Professor
Department of Biochemistry
Aligarh Muslim University
Aligarh, Uttar Pradesh, India

Foreword

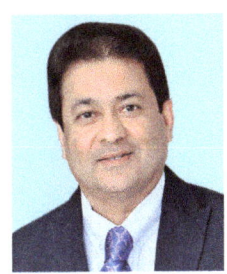

It is an extreme honor and delight to write a foreword for the book entitled *Clinical Focus on Male and Female Infertility*. This book has been compiled and beautifully edited by Dr Narendra Malhotra, Dr Jaideep Malhotra, Dr Neharika Malhotra, Dr Keshav Malhotra, and Dr Shaheen Anjum. Contributions of the highest academic standards and excellence have been made by renowned Infertility Specialists from all over India. The author list is a thrilling mixture of reputed researchers, clinicians and embryologists from over the country.

Congratulations are in order for the brilliant Editors for such a complete book on male and female infertility. The book gives the reader a background, the diagnostic evaluation and work-up of infertile couples as well as the options of all the modern ART options.

Over the past few years, formidable progress has been made in the fields of Reproductive Biology, Endocrinology, Ultrasound in Infertility and Assisted Reproductive Technologies. Reproductive medicine has been refined, modified and has now entered a new era carrying great promises of rapid advancement and opening of new horizons for the infertile couple.

The book has comprehensive and in-depth coverage of all aspects of infertility management such as evaluation of the infertile couple, the intricacies of male factor infertility and sperm integrity, the association of environment, genetics and nutrition in infertility, ultrasound evaluation and the management of anovulatory and unexplained infertility. It also covers the various ART methods of IUI, IVF, ICSI and third party reproduction.

My best wishes to all those who have been associated with the publishing of this book.

Jatin P Shah
MBBS MD DGO FICOG
Director
Mumbai Fertility Centre
IVF Specialist
Mumbai, Maharashtra, India

Preface

WHO estimates the overall prevalence of primary infertility in India to be between 3.9 and 16.8%, this translates around 50 lakh couples suffering from infertility. Research has shown that psychological distress and physical abuse is significantly more common in infertile women than in their fertile counterparts.

To bring the smile on faces of these couples, we have to do proper evaluation and management.

The diagnostic evaluation and management should be conducted in a systematic, expeditious, and cost-effective manner to identify all relevant factors, with an initial emphasis on the least invasive methods for the detection of the most common causes of infertility. The pace and extent of evaluation should take into account the couple's preferences, patient age, the duration of infertility, and the unique features of the medical history and physical examination.

This book is a part of *Clinical Focus Series* which provide overview of evaluation and management of infertile couple. It is a comprehensive and easy reference book which provide the practical tips for undergraduates, postgraduates and healthcare workers.

In producing series of handbooks and practical manuals, the editors and authors sincerely hope that the healthcare professionals and trainees will benefit and provide better care to infertile couples.

Neharika Malhotra
Jaideep Malhotra
Narendra Malhotra
Shaheen Anjum
Keshav Malhotra

Acknowledgments

We have the pleasure of introducing *Clinical Focus on Male and Female Infertility*.

We thank the Almighty God for helping us throughout the journey of completing this task. Our heartfelt gratitude to Dr Jatin P Shah for accepting to write the foreword for this book and also give his blessings.

It is with utmost pleasure that we thank Dr Narendra Malhotra and Dr Jaideep Malhotra, our mentors and guide for this Clinical Series, who lent their considerable clinical and academic prowess. Their enthusiasm and encouragement kept us motivated to accomplish this task.

In constructing a compilation of this breadth, clinicians from several departments and their expertise were needed to add vital, contemporaneous information. We wish to thank all our contributors who responded to our requests with promptness. Our heartfelt thanks to them.

We wish to appreciate the efforts of M/s Jaypee Brothers Medical Publishers (P) Ltd, New Delhi, India for bringing out this book in its final shape with their talent of skillfully and expediently coordinating and overseeing composition. We also thank publishing team of M/s Jaypee Brothers Medical Publishers, especially Ms Rajni Chauhan. Without the thoughtful, creative efforts of many, our *Clinical Focus Series* would have been a barren wasteland of words. Their attention to detail and accurate renderings added important academic support to our words.

Our special appreciation and thanks to all our colleagues, friends who supported our idea of bringing out this series and gave us the confidence to finish this book. Lastly, we offer an enthusiastic thanks to our families and friends. Without their patience, generosity and encouragement, this task would have been impossible. We sincerely thank you for your love and support which kept us going to finish this work of ours.

Editors
Shaheen Anjum
Keshav Malhotra

Contents

1. **Evaluation of Infertile Couple** 1
   Shikha Seth, Narendra Malhotra

2. **Male Infertility** 10
   Deeba Khanam, Shaheen Anjum, Keshav Malhotra

3. **The Environment and Infertility** 16
   Jaya Sharma, Jaideep Malhotra, Divya Yadav

4. **Genetics and Infertility** 22
   Ruchika Garg, Rekha Rani

5. **Nutrition and Infertility** 25
   Sufia Naseem, Shaheen Anjum

6. **Ultrasound Evaluation of Infertility** 33
   Maneesha Jain, Narendra Malhotra

7. **Management of Tubal Factor in Fertility** 46
   Anu Agarwal, Shikha Sachan

8. **Anovulatory Infertility** 52
   Rehana Najam, Jaideep Malhotra

9. **Unexplained Infertility** 61
   Neharika Malhotra, Narendra Malhotra

10. **Assisted Reproductive Techniques: When to Refer** 68
    Saeeda Wasim, Sharique Ahmad

Index *77*

CHAPTER 1

Evaluation of Infertile Couple

Shikha Seth, Narendra Malhotra

INTRODUCTION

Infertility in itself is a vast subject because both male and female partner-related factors are responsible for successful conception which we need to identify first for helping them to conceive. From an evaluation point of view, infertility is divided into two groups: Primary and Secondary, and each into subgroups—Male and Female, which are further subdivided for stepwise strategic workup **(Fig. 1)**. Few factors/causes are modifiable or treatable and few are not. Cases, where no gross factor or cause is identifiable on strategic basic workup, are termed as unexplained infertility and thus it is the diagnosis of exclusion. With the advent and rapid advancement of artificial reproductive techniques (ART) researchers have found various ways for helping couples with unexplained infertility or where no correctable measures are available. In another way, we can say, for successful infertility management it is utmost required to know the factors responsible and ways

---

Infertility Basic Evaluation
<35 years: 12 months after plan
>35 years 6 months after
>40 years or symptomatics—expedited

Detailed History of Couple
- Duration of infertility
- Menstrual history
- H/o past pregnancy
- Sexual history
- Personal history
- Medical/drug history
- H/o pelvic surgical
- H/o trauma, tumor, TB
- Contraceptive history
- H/o infection—RTI/STIs
- Occupational hazards
- Dietary history

Detailed examination
- Thyroid and breast
- Per-abdomen, local
- Per-speculum
- Bimanual examination

Investigations: →

Male Factor
1. Semen analysis
   Assessment by WHO criteria mentioned in **Box 1**
   Sperm function, male endocrine, immunological, genetic tests are not 1st line tests

Female Factor
1. *Ovarian factors:*
   - Ovulation testing
   - Ovarian reserve
2. *Uterine factor:*
   - Structural anomalies—USG-TVS
   Implantation related Doppler, UBPP not 1st line
3. *Tubal factor—patency:*
   - HSG, SSG, HyCoSy,
   Endoscopic tests are not 1st line
4. *Endocrine factor:*
   - Thyroid and day 21—progesterone
   LH, FSH, prolactin, insulin, estrogen leptin, SHBG are not 1st line tests

Fig. 1: Infertility basic evaluation.

to identify them with a detailed history and strategic investigations. This chapter is focused on the basic initial evaluation to help any gynecology practitioner when a couple reports to his/her outpatient department wanting the pregnancy.

When to Start Work-up for Infertility?

- As per the definition, infertility is being diagnosed on failure to conceive after one complete year of regular unprotective sexual activity.
  - After one year, if the female partner's age is less than 35 years while
  - It may be started in six months trial if the female partner is 35 or older.
- Secondly, if there is any genuine medical/surgical reason to suspect an underlying problem in history, the workup should be started earlier, for example if a female is having menstrual cycle irregularity or a male is having an erectile disorder.

Indications for Immediate or Expedited Evaluation

- Oligomenorrhea, amenorrhea, irregular cycles, intermenstrual bleeding
- Known or suspected peritoneal, tubal or uterine pathology, endometriosis (stage III and IV)
- Suspected male factor infertility
- Sexual dysfunction
- Genetic, familial disorder or acquired conditions affecting fertility.

Starting of Infertility Evaluation

Both partners are to be evaluated simultaneously, but if required individual focused interview separately may be opted for especially with sexual activity, performance, erection, ejaculation, timing, frequency, and any difficulties faced.

Detailed History of Couple

- Should be taken in a comfortable environment
- Duration of infertility and check for results of previous evaluation/treatment
- Menstrual history detail for assessing ovulation, molimina, mittelschmerz
- Pregnancy history and outcome in case of secondary infertility (abortion, ectopic, biochemical, unknown location)
- *Sexual history:* Frequency, timing, interests, problems faced, libido, erectile/ejaculatory dysfunction, or any pain (dyspareunia, vaginismus)
- Personal history (addictions and habits)
- Medical/drug history, past pelvic surgical history, and trauma,
- Contraceptive history, reproductive tract infections (RTIs)/sexually transmitted infections (STIs)
- Occupational exposure or other environmental hazards
- Dietary history especially those with abnormal BMI
- Usually, it is multifactorial so all subgroups be given equal importance.

Counseling

Infertile couples must be briefly sensitized about the reproductive system through models or charts to make them understand the need for the tests and their timings.

■ MALE FACTOR EVALUATION

Detail history of male partner to be taken.

Physical examination of male is only to be performed if there is any history suggestive of pathological problem or any abnormality in semen analysis. Male partner should be examined for secondary sexual characters, an inspection of penis, urethral opening, and prepuce. Palpation of the scrotum for testes size (Average 15 mL), consistency and tenderness, cystic malformations, or thickening of epididymis and vas and hernia, hydroceles or lymphoceles, varicocele, lymphadenopathy should be noted. Finally, the prostate is palpated by rectal digital examination. Seminal vesicles are normally not palpable until they are congested or diseased.

The single primary test for the evaluation of male infertility is the "semen analysis": Couple should refrain from sexual intercourse 3-5 days before sample collection for the best results as the period of continence preceding collection has a remarkable effect on sperm concentration and motility. Sample should be collected through masturbation in a sterile wide-mouthed container, preferably in the clinic itself so that it can be processed in one hour.

Semen Analysis[1,2]

Color: Whitish grey normally. Discoloration hints towards infection. The red tinge suggests the presence of blood in semen and indicates either trauma, inflammation or tumor of the genital tract.

Odor: Usually should be odorless.

Liquefaction: Immediately after ejaculation semen coagulates and subsequently liquefies in 20-40 minutes. Lack of coagulation indicates agenesis of seminal vesicles or obstruction of ejaculatory ducts. If the coagulum fails to liquefy, this is probably due to a lack of prostatic lytic enzymes. Persistent coagulum traps sperms and restricts motility.

Consistency: Following liquefaction semen takes a viscous consistency. Hyperviscosity is checked by pouring it into another jar and observing its ability to fractionate.

Volume: Normal volume is 2-5 mL. Semen volume is contributed by seminal vesicles. Seminal plasma functions as a vehicle, diluent, nutrient, and buffering medium protecting sperm from hostile vaginal pH. Reduced volume can be because of incomplete ejaculation, occlusion of the ejaculatory duct, or androgen deficiency. Inflammation is responsible for hyperspermia (>10 mL) and resultant dilution of cell content.

BOX 1: World Health Organization (WHO) normal semen parameters.

Volume	2–5 mL
pH	7.2–7.8
Color	homogeneous greyish white
Consistency	Leave pipette as discrete droplets
Liquefaction	30–60 minutes
Fructose	>1200 ng/mL
Sperm concentration	>20 million/mL
Total count	Min 40 million/ejaculate
Motility	50% or more with forward progression or 25% or more with rapid linear progression in 1st hr
Morphology	>30% or more with normal forms or 15% or more with Tygerberg strict criteria
Vitality	50% or more
Leukocytes	Fewer than 1 million/mL
Dead forms	<10%

pH: Below 7 (acidic) suggests either occlusion of ejaculatory ducts, contamination with urine, chronic inflammation, or infection of accessory sex glands.

Microscopy of Semen

- On microscopy, if agglutination is found and more than 10% of sperms show agglutination, infection or immunological problems should be suspected.
- If no sperm is seen, then it is termed 'Azoospermia' while 'Aspermia' describes where no seminal fluid is discharged during orgasm.
- *Sperm count and concentration* is determined with help of a Hemocytometer, Makler or Neubauer chamber, or electronic counting as a Coulter counter.
- Sperm concentration is expressed as a number of sperms per milliliter while

Total sperm count = Sperm concentration x semen volume

Fertilizing capacity is affected if sperm concentration. Is below 20×10^6 /mL? The critical limit is 5×10^6/mL, where IVF outcome is also poor and ideally opted for ICSI.

Sperm Motility

Three parameters are assessed in this regard: (1) Percentage of motile cells; (2) Type of motility; and (3) Maintenance of motility as a function of time. Motility loss is expected 10–20% within 3 hours. Normal ejaculate has 25% rapid linear and 50% fast progressive spermatozoa. The usual speed of sperm is 25 micron/sec or 3 mm/hour.

"Asthenozoospermia" where motile cell percentage is below 50% on 100 sperm cell examination in Makler chamber. In an era of automated semen analysis, computer-assisted semen analysis (CASA) offers the advantage of standardization, quality control, and research point of view.

Sperm Viability

All non-movers are not dead sperms. Vitality is checked by supravital staining. Eosin which does not penetrate living cells so-stained cells are diagnosed as dead. The presence of dead forms is termed "Necrozoospermia". Viable but non-motile sperm hints toward immotile cilia syndrome.

BOX 2: ACOG and ASRM recommendations.[19,20]

- Infertility evaluation may be offered to patients who by definition has infertility or at high risk of it
- Older females (>35 years) should get an expedited evaluation and treatment after 6 months of failed attempts. In case of those above 40 years, more immediate evaluation be warranted.
- Comprehensive medical history including relevant points of infertility etiology be obtained from couple.
- Targeted physical examination be performed in female and its reasonable to refer the male partner to specialist having expertise in male reproductive medicine.
- Investigations of female should focus on ovarian reserve, ovulatory function and structural abnormality.
- Imaging be used for tubal patency, pelvic pathology and assessing ovarian reserve. HSG or SHG are recommended tests for tubal patency.
- Advanced tests as laparoscopy, MRI, karyotype, immunological, sperm function, genetic evaluation should not be routinely ordered. Hormonal tests as Estradiol, Prolactin, FSH, LH, Inhibin B, Clomiphene challenge test, Testosterone, etc. be done only when suggestive history is there.

(ACOG: American College of Obstetricians and Gynecologists; ASRM: American Society of Reproductive Medicine; FSH: follicle stimulating hormone; HSG: hysterosalpingogram; LH: Luteinizing hormone; SHG: sonohysterogram)

Sperm Morphology

Typical spermatozoa has a head, neck, midpiece, principal piece, and tail. About 4% normal forms are the lowest limit below which fertility is unlikely to even with ART while the upper limit of the grey zone is chosen at 45% normal forms. More than 70% of abnormal morphology in the ejaculate is considered "Teratozoospermia".

Special Tests for Abnormal Examination/Semen Report and Unexplained Infertility

Biochemical tests include markers of the functionality of secondary sex glands and their products which might affect the fertilization capacity of sperm-like fructose (energy source) and coagulable protein from the seminal vesicle, liquifying enzymes from the prostate. Fructose is measured by chromatography and value of 1200 ng/mL is considered normal.

Sperm function tests is opted in the cases of all normal parameter semen with unexplained infertility, where it becomes important to check the efficacy of sperm in vaginal environment in-vitro" based on immunological factors and responsible for IVF failure too.[3]

Hormonal tests are usually done when concentration and motility are extremely poor. *Testosterone* and *FSH* are tested to differentiate testicular and HPO axis defects.

Testicular biopsy helps diagnose the obstruction in case of azoospermia/aspermia.

Note:
- Urine analysis helps diagnose retrograde ejaculation.
- A single report showing abnormal sperm count, concentration or motility should ideally be repeated after 3 weeks and 3 months.
- Special tests should not be routinely ordered under basic evaluation.

■ FEMALE FACTOR EVALUATION

Start with detailed menstrual, contraception, coital, sexual history, general, systemic, pelvic examination, and further evaluation is subcategorized into 4 sections. All sections both anatomical and functional factors affect fertility.

Physical Examination

Height, weight, BMI, blood pressure, pulse, temperature, thyroid (enlargement, nodularity or tenderness), breast (size, tanner stage, nipple discharge), hirsutism, pubic and axillary hair, local genital examination, per speculum examination for abnormality or discharge, pelvic bimanual examination (noting uterus size, shape, position, mobility, adnexal, and cul-de-sac tenderness, organomegaly, mass).

1. Uterine Factor

a. *Cervix:* Pre-ovulatory mucous is watery in consistency, copious in amount, acellular and shows 'Spinnbarkeit' (stretchability) and 'Ferning' to allow sperms to pass in easily and defines the "Cervical Score". In 3–5% of cases, it is the cervix responsible for infertility if scarred, stenosed due to previous surgeries (LEEP, cone biopsy, electrocautery) or D&C or secondary to infection of endocervical glands or congenital defect. Immunological factors are tested by anti-sperm antibodies and by SCMC and SPT as mentioned above.

b. *Uterine corpus:* Anatomical defects such as cavitary adhesion, endometrial polyps, myoma, adenomyosis, septum, or other congenital malformations and functionally as nonresponsive, thin endometrium with integrin deficiency are the points which are assessed by Imaging (USG), HSG and SSG (for cavitary filling defects).[4] Transvaginal sonography with Doppler is the best measure for endometrial assessment at ovulatory or implantation time as well as differentiating the endometrial/sub-endometrial/myometrial entities.[5]

3D-sonography, MRI—for structural defects and direct visualization of cavity by hysteroscopy and guided biopsy for integrin assay are the advanced tests to be done selectively in case-to-case basis not as first line evaluation until suspected by history or examination.[6]

2. Tubal Factor

Tube is a fine and delicate structure and we do not have any good tests for its functionality as peristalsis and ciliary movement. Tubal factor is most common cause of infertility among female factors. Nowadays water-based contrast dyes are preferred as compared to earlier oil ones. Pushing the contrast with some force itself used to improve fertility as they removes the fine plugs and obstructions.[7] Hysterosalpingogram (HSG) has its advantage that reveals the internal architecture of uterine and tubal lumen which no other patency test gives.

Sono-salpingography (SSG) is minimal invasive technique and avoids X-ray exposure. It does not differentiate between uni/bilateral patency.

HyCoSy: Hystero-contrast sonography is another adjunct which determines the patency with contrast agent with air bubbles to aid in identification of medium as it passes through tubes with higher accuracy then SSG using transvaginal scan.[8]

Although the laparoscopic chromo-pertubation is considered as a gold-standard test but should not be considered as first line or basic evaluation part as it is invasive test. Laparoscopic direct visualization gives the advantage of peritubal disease identification, and adhesiolysis then and there is possible, if required.

Falloposcopy and salpingoscopy are two advanced tests for evaluation of tubal lumen.[9] Laparoscopy has the advantage of direct identification of pelvic disorders, a biopsy can be collected from peritubular adhesions (infective or endometriotic), and possibility of surgical correction of blocked tubes can be materialized.

3. Ovarian Factor

Ovary is the store/reservoir of gametocytes which continues to deplete over time. The function is indirectly assessed by regular 28–30 days of menstrual cycles.

Serum progesterone obtained 1 week prior to the expected menstrual cycle is the best policy rather than fixing to the policy of day 21. Value above 3 ng/mL provides presumptive evidence of ovulation.

Antral follicle count (AFC): Less than 5–7 follicles at baseline D2-D4 USG is poor. Too many AFC more than 10–12 are seen in PCOS which is responsible for poor infertility outcome.

Follicular monitoring: Folliculogenesis can be analyzed directly by sonographic follicular growth and rupture monitoring, while ovulation is evaluated either by serum progesterone levels (Day 21-24) or secretary changes in the premenstrual endometrial sampling.

Anti-Müllerian hormone (AMH) is derived from granulosa cells of pre- and antral follicles and is a marker of ovarian reserve. Low (as in poor ovarian reserve) and high (as in PCOS) levels both affect folliculogenesis. Value less than 1 ng/mL suggest poor reserve. S. AMH is surrogate for antral follicle count for PCOS cases.[15]

FSH: Done between Day 2–5 of menstrual cycle, if more than 10 IU/mL suggest poor reserve. Women with poor reserve or high FSH before age of 40 years she should be evaluated for fragile X carrier screening—FMR1 pre-mutations.

Endometrial sampling using the Pipelle or the thin cannula in premenstrual phase (around Day 22–25 in 28–30 day cycle) and histology for confirmation of ovulation by presence of secretory changes is also an option and can be done as an OPD procedure. Endometrial biopsy using metal Curette's should preferably be avoided. The sampling procedure steps also hints about the cervical canal related abnormalities if any (steonosis).

Ovulation predictor kits for testing LH in the urine samples in mid-cycle but their reliability, accuracy is poor and have high false results. Patients with PCOS have high basal level of LH in whole cycle and give false-positive results.

4. Endocrine Factor

Apart from the functional HPO-axis, endocrine glands have to function synergistically to have fertility as thyroid, adrenals, etc.

Other hormonal evaluations be done only when the history or examination is suggestive. HPO axis evaluation is done by baseline D2/3 levels of FSH and LH. Prolactin is the hormone that in excess affects the HPO axis as well as ovaries directly resulting in abnormal cycles and steroidogenesis. Some physiological aspects such as improper sleep and stress also affect it and are seen in association with hypothyroidism which needs to be evaluated and treated first. Research have found role of prolactin and other endocrine micro-environment on human antral follicle development.[10, 11]

Thyroid evaluation and luteal progesterone (D 21) are considered under basic evaluation of infertility. Both hypo- and hyperthyroidism affect fertility and therefore be tested by TSH, T3 and T4, and antithyroid antibodies when values are grossly abnormal or clinical findings are suggestive.[12]

■ IN UNEXPLAINED CASES

Active free circulating levels of most of the above hormones depend on the sex-hormone binding globulin (SHBG). If SHBG is low, even at normal total hormonal level prominent effects are seen due to higher levels of free sex hormones. Leptin a hormone from adipose tissue has key role in regulating energy uptake and metabolism. Increased leptin affects LH pulsatility, impaired follicular growth, and anovulation[13]

Hyperinsulinemia and insulin resistance is responsible for anovulation in PCOS cases and is seen in association with hyperandrogenism due to adrenal hormones. Hyperandrogenism presents as acne, hirsutism, amenorrhea and at a higher level as features of virilization as hoarse voice, enlargement of clitoris, and temporal balding evaluated by DHEAS, androstenedione (adrenal), testosterone (ovaries theca cells) testing.[14]

Ultrasonography—Transvaginal (TVS) has a special role in the evaluation of infertility and in all subcategories so requires a special mention for comprehensive assessment and interpretation of fertility aspects, starting from the gateway cervix. TVS can define cervicitis, presence of Nabothian cysts, internal os, or stenosis. In uterus, it can identify all structural anomalies acquired (myoma, adenomyosis, polyp), cavitary lesions by saline infusion (SIS), and other pelvic pathologies (endometrioma, ovarian cysts). Evaluation of endometrium by its thickness and pattern (homogeneous or triple line).

Tubal evaluation is supported by "Sonosalpingography" (SSG) where saline is pushed through the Foley's no 8 in uterine cavity and flow, spillage, and collection in the Pouch of Douglas suggests the patency. HyCoSy is also known as "Contrast Sono-hystero-salpingography" (HyCoSy) where Echovist a USG contrast media is instilled through Foley's no. 8.

Ovarian size, echotexture (PCOS), follicular development, prediction of ovulation (anechoic area-double contour, irregularity of follicular lining), confirmation of ovulation (loss of dominant follicle, crenated/hemorrhagic corpus luteum and newly appearing fluid in pouch) are possible on TVS.

TVS is useful noninvasive tool for antral follicle count (AFC-D2-D4) later follicular monitoring and endometrial phasic assessment as thickness and pattern of proliferative (triple line with the thick outer line reaching 8-10 mm), luteal phase (homogeneous hyperechoic) which helps in assessing and predicting the outcome too in the hands of gynecologist.[16]

Color Doppler has facilitated in understanding the physiology and predicting the implantation probability, most popular being "Applebaum score" which measures contractions of endomyometrial junction, uterine artery pulsatility index (PI), endometrial and myometrial flow along with the endometrial thickness and zonal layering. Pulsatility index (PI) measurement in ovarian, uterine artery, perifollicular and endometrial vascularity can help in predicting ovulation and receptivity respectively. Uterine biophysical scoring is not the routine baseline infertility evaluation test and being utilized only for unexplained infertility, implantation failure cases.[17,18]

Ovulation induction-associated complications and ART procedures such as oocyte retrieval and embryo transfer also require sonographic expertise.

■ CONCLUSION

Treatment of infertility is a team approach involving gynecologist, endocrinologist, andrologist, urologists and ART lab experts and comprehensive workup of couple. Couple counseling, giving them true information and removing their anxiety is important for successful results or stepping ahead in evaluation if primary workup is normal. In general practice, instead of prescribing the whole battery of tests at time at initial phase, it is always better to go step by step from those factors which are suspected to be affected based on history and examination shown in **Figure 1**. For regular menstrual cycle cases (21-35 days), additional testing for ovulation is not required, until there is other findings on examination. Both male and female assessment be done simultaneously.

■ REFERENCES

1. WHO Laboratory Manual for the Examination of Human Semen and Sperm: Cervical Mucous Interaction, 4th edition. Cambridge Univ Press, 1999
2. Lundquest F, et al. Aspects of the biochemistry of human semen. Acta Physiologica Scnadinavica. 1949;19(Suppl 66):7-105.

3. Kremer J. The immunology of cervical sterility: its assessment and management. Contracept Fertil Sex (Paris). 1979;7(2):141-6.
4. Gordts S, Brosens JJ, Fusi L, Benagiano G, Brosne I. Uterine adenomyosis: a need for uniform terminology and consensus classification. Reprod Biomed Online. 2008: 17(2):244-8.
5. Tocci A, Greco E, Ubaldi FM. Adenomyosis and endometrial-sub-endometrial myometrium unit disruption disease are two different entities. Reprod Biomed Online. 2008;17(2):281-91.
6. Golan A, et al. Diagnostic hysteroscocpy: its value in an IVF-ET unit. Fertil Steril. 1992;58:1237-9.
7. De Cherny AH, Kort H, et al. Increased pregnancy rate with oil soluble hysterosalpingography. Fertil Steril. 1980;33:407
8. Diechert U, Schlief R, Van de Sandt M, Juhnke. Transvaginal HyCoSy compared with conventional tubal diagnostics. Human Reproduction. 1989;4:418-24.
9. Henry, Suchet J. Endoscopy of the tube. Acta Eur Fertil. 1985;16:139.
10. Kaupilla, A et al. Hyperprolactinemia and ovarian function. Fertil Steril. 1988;49:437.
11. Mc Natty KP, et al. The relationship between plasma prolactin and the endocrine microenvironment of the developing human antral follicle. Fertil Steril. 1979;32:43.
12. Krassas GE. Thyroid disease and female reproduction. Fertil Steril. 2000;74(6): 1063-70.
13. Agrawal SK, Vogel K, Weitsman SR, Magoffin DA. Leptin antagonizes IGF-1 augmentation of steroidogenesis in granulosa and theca cells of the human ovary J. Clin Endocrin and Metabol. 1999;84:1072-6.
14. Dunaif A, et al. Insulin resistance and the polycystic ovary syndrome: mechanism and implication for pathogenesis. Endocr Rev. 1997;18:774-800.
15. Pigny P, Jonard S, Robert Y, Dewailly D. Sreum AMH as a surrogate for antral follicle count for definition of PCOS. J Clin Endocrinol Metab. 2006;91:941-5.
16. Hackeloer BJ, Fleming R, Robinson HP, et al. Correlation of ultrasonic and endocrinologic assessment of human follicular development. Am J Obstet Gynecol. 1979;135:122.
17. Applebaum M. The Uterine Biophysical Profile (UBP) in endo-sonography in obstetrics and gynaecology. Allahabadia G (Ed) Rotunda Medical Technologies Ltd, Mumbai. 1997;343-52.
19. ACOG committee opinion: infertility workup for women health specialists.2019 https://www.acog.org/clinical/clinical-guidance/committee-opinion/articles/2019/06/infertility-workup-for-the-womens-health-specialist
20. Fertility Evaluation of Infertile Women: a committee opinion (Practice Committee of ASRM) Fertility and Sterility.® 2021;116(5): 0015-0282.

Male Infertility

Deeba Khanam, Shaheen Anjum, Keshav Malhotra

■ INTRODUCTION

Infertility is defined as inability to conceive after 1 year of regular sexual intercourse without using any contraception.[1] Various bodies like World Health Organization (WHO), the American Society for Reproductive Medicine and American Medical Association (AMA) have labeled it as a disease which requires evaluation and treatment.[2] The couples, who could not conceive in the first year of married life contribute to approximately 15% and majority of them conceive in second year of regular unprotected sexual intercourse. A male factor as an isolated cause for infertility is present in 20% of infertile couples and may exist along with other causes of infertility in approximately 30-40%[3] of infertile population. Infertility evaluation is recommended after 1 year of failed attempt to conceive, however it should be proposed after 6 months when the age of female partner is greater than 35 years of age.[4]

■ MALE INFERTILITY

Definition

Primary male infertility is defined as a condition where male has never been able to contribute to a clinical pregnancy, whereas secondary male infertility refers to a condition where the male partner is unable to impregnate her sexual partner, but who had procreated a clinical pregnancy previously.[2]

Causes

The causes of male infertility can be identified as factors acting at pre-testicular, testicular or post-testicular level.[5] However, despite advancements 50% causes cannot be clinically identified and labeled as idiopathic infertility.

Pretesticular Causes

They are known as extra-gonadal endocrine disorders originating in the pituitary, hypothalamus or adrenals. A systemic problem could progress from hormonal imbalances, genetic disorders, poor health, obesity, dietary and age patterns.

Hypogonadotropic hypogonadism:
- Idiopathic
- Kallmann syndrome, Prader-Willi syndrome, Laurence-Moon-Biedl syndrome

Pituitary causes:
- Prolactinoma
- Isolated LH deficiency
- Isolated FSH deficiency
- Craniopharyngioma
- Pituitary tumors
- Infiltrative diseases
- Trauma
- Critical and chronic diseases

Coital disorders:
- Erectile dysfunction
- Ejaculatory disorder

Testicular disorders:
- Varicocele
- Cryptorchidism
- Noonan syndrome
- Vanishing testicular disease
- Myotonic dystrophy
- Y-chromosome microdeletion
- XX male (sex reversal syndrome)
- XYY male
- Noonan syndrome (male Turner syndrome)
- Androgen receptor defect

Testicular injury:
- Trauma
- Torsion

Systemic diseases:
- Liver diseases
- Renal diseases
- Congenital adrenal hyperplasia (CAH)
- Alcoholism
- HIV
- Orchitis
- Obesity
- Chronic gastroenteritis
- Hematological diseases

Gonadotoxins:
- Radiotherapy
- Drugs
- Toxins.

Post-testicular Causes
- Obstruction
- Transportation and ductal system defects
- *Congenital:* Diethylstilbestrol (DES) exposure, cystic fibrosis
- *Acquired:* Infections, surgery, stone, prostatic cyst, antisperm antibodies
- Immotile cilia syndrome Ejaculation defects
- Diabetes, bladder neck surgery, colon, rectal, prostate surgery, spinal cord injury
- Infections.

Evaluation

Evaluation of infertility requires simultaneous assessment of both male and female partners. The American Urological Association (AUA) and American Society of Reproductive Medicine (ASRM) recommends that at a minimum, the infertility work-up includes a detailed history, physical examination and two separate semen analyses to identify risk factors for male infertility.[6] The consistent presence of abnormal semen parameters supports meticulous evaluation of male partner furthermore. Semen parameters are assessed according to WHO 5th edition recommendations[1] as mentioned in **Table 1**.

TABLE 1: Semen parameters (WHO 5th Edition recommendations).

Semen Parameter	One-sided lower reference limit (Fifth centiles with 95% confidence intervals)
Semen volume	1.5 mL (1.4–1.7)
Total sperm number	39 million per ejaculate (33–46)
Sperm concentration	15 million/mL (12–16 million/mL)
Vitality	58% Live (55–63%)
Progressive motility	32% (31–34%)
Total motility (Progressive + Non-progressive)	40%
Morphologically normal forms	4.0% (3.0–4.0)

The evaluation of men with abnormal SAs and/or abnormal reproductive history, including physical examination and selected laboratory and radiologic assessment, should be done by expert in male infertility.

History

While evaluating the male partner with detailed history (reproductive, sexual, past, personal and family) and meticulous physical examination[7] of male reproductive organs existing or newly diagnosed comorbid conditions are identified, e.g. diabetes, endocrinopathies, hypertension, etc., and treatment is offered as increasing number of studies report increased medical comorbidities associated with abnormal SA.[8]

Physical Examination

- It includes general and local examinations.
- Body habitus—eunuchoid body, infantile hair, poor muscular development, longer lower body—endocrine disorders
- Truncal obesity, striae, Moon facies—Cushing syndrome
- Thyroid swelling
- Hepatomegaly, lymph nodes for lymphomas.

Local Examination

- *Phallus:* Meatal location as hypospadias/epispadias, penile lesions/ulcers/discharge
- *Scrotum/testes:* Examination for previous scars, position, size and consistency of the testes and palpation of testicular masses.
- *Epididymides:* Size, shape and consistency to be evaluated. Exclusion of induration/dilation which suggests obstruction.
- *Vas deferens:* Examination of its presence, shape/consistency as its abnormality may be suggestive of CFTR mutation.
- *Digital rectal examination:* Evaluation of prostatic cysts or dilated seminal vesicles to rule out EDO (epididymal obstruction).

Semen Analysis (SA)

Individual semen parameters measured in the SA are not diagnostic of male infertility, however isolated parameters like azoospermia, necrozoospermia or specific type of morphological pattern like globozoospermia may raise fertility concerns.[6] ASRM states that an endocrine evaluation is not indicated as first line investigation but is vindicated with clinical findings suggestive of endocrinopathy, sexual dysfunction (decreased libido, erectile dysfunction) and abnormal laboratory parameters such as oligozoospermia or azoospermia are obtained.[8] Endocrinal evaluation includes testing for free testosterone, LH, FSH, and prolactin levels in men evaluated for male sexual dysfunction.

Oligozoospermia/Oligospermia (Decreased Sperm Count)

Oligospermia (<10 million sperm/mL) in semen analysis requires hormonal evaluation of the male partner (FSH, testosterone and luteinizing hormone) and is also indicated in men with sexual dysfunction. Low serum testosterone (<300 ng/dL) warrants PRL levels evaluation to exclude hypo- gonadotropic hypogonadism in men.[9]

Azoospermia (Absence of Sperm in Ejaculate)

This finding warrants classifying azoospermia into obstructive and non-obstructive type. On the basis of history, physical examination and hormonal studies this differentiation can be made. Men with azoospermia and normal semen volume, smaller testes on examination and elevated FSH levels are suggestive of testicular failure and will have NOA (azoospermia due to impaired sperm production). Men with azoospermia with decreased semen volume (<0.5 or 1.0 mL), normal testicular size (e.g., testis length >4.6 cm), and normal FSH levels (<7.6) suffer from obstructive azoospermia, especially when supported by physical examination of proximal epididymis enlargement and absent vas deferens.[9]

Severe Oligospermia (Less than 5 Million Count) and Non-obstructive Azoospermia

Men with severe oligospermia (<5 M/mL) including NOA should be evaluated with karyotyping and Y-microdeletion studies.[10] The most common chromosomal abnormality is Klinefelter syndrome (47 XXY), and second most common genetic cause is Y-chromosome microdeletions of azoospermic genes. Sperms may be retrieved through microsurgical sperm extraction in the former and may not be retrieved at all in specific Y- chromosome microdeletions.

Obstructive Azoospermia

Diagnosis is suggested by azoospermia, normal FSH and testosterone levels and physical examinations confirming absence of vas deferens, epididymal obstruction or ejaculatory duct obstruction. If congenital absence of vas deferens is suspected, unilateral or bilateral, then *CFTR* gene mutation evaluation should be advised in the male partner and if found to be positive female partner should be screened for the presence of carrier gene which may possibly affect the transmission of the defect to the offspring.[11,12] These mutations are also associated with renal abnormalities and therefore transrectal ultrasound is advised for confirmation of diagnosis and proper counseling. Treatment incudes extraction of sperm through different microsurgical techniques. Reversible causes of obstructive azoospermia should be treated as per the norms.

Asthenozoospermia (Decreased Sperm Motility)

Specific movement attributes (average path velocity, moving straight, and amplitude of lateral sperm head displacement) of spermatozoa are considered features of semen quality that can facilitate cervical barrier penetration.[13] The causes of asthenozoospermia include varicocele, genetic abnormalities, lifestyle, radiations, infections, psychological stress, and environmental factors. Assessing the factors responsible and preventing or regulating them may affect the motility. Researchers have proposed certain novel motility enhancing proteins derived from caprine serum which are known to enhance sperm motility in vitro.[14,15] However, ART has been proposed for abnormalities in sperm motility for now.

Sperm Vitality

It is an important predictor of sperm viability and is estimated by percentage of live spermatozoa with intact membranes. WHO 2010 guidelines states that 42% dead sperm is the cut-off for necrospermia (dead sperm) and 58% should be live (viable). DNA fragmentation is the last step of sperm death and is linked to poor sperm viability. Both increased DNA fragmentation and poor viability have positive correlation with male infertility and the parameters are influenced by number of systemic and local conditions associated with males[16] and that needs identification. However DNA fragmentation studies are not proposed as first line in initial evaluation of male infertility but may be used in RPL and for sperm selection in ART.[9]

Pyospermia

If the round cells on SA are increased in number (>1 million/mL), then attempts should be made to further to differentiate white blood cells (pyospermia) from germ cells. Semen culture is recommended in patients with pyospermia.[9]

Postejaculatory Urine Analysis

This test should be considered to identify retrograde ejaculation and differentiate it from obstructive causes of oligo/azoospermia. When the volume of ejaculate is less (<2 mL), condition is known as hypospermia or if there is no ejaculate at all, known as aspermia.[1] Abstinence of 1 day or less or loss of sample can be the contributory factor. To evaluate urine sample, it should be centrifuged for 10 minutes at 300 rpm and seen at 400 magnification.[17] Any sperm in urine is diagnostic of retrograde ejaculation.

Imaging

Imaging is not used as initial investigating modality in male infertility evaluation.[9] The main role of imaging is to identify the cause of infertility and help categorize it into Obstructive and non-obstructive causes. When the examination of scrotum is difficult to, especially in obesity and then scrotal ultrasound may be advised. Testicular atrophy, varicocele, absence of vas deferens and dysplastic seminal vesicles may be identified through sonography,[18,19] when examination findings are unable to determine the pathology. Ejaculatory duct anomalies require TRUS (Transrectal ultrasonography) for diagnosis.[20]

Management

Successful pregnancy requires a sperm which is morphologically and functionally normal and therefore male infertility requires assiduous evaluation. ART has opened opportunities for infertile couples with subtle and apparent male factor infertility. Treatment offered is case based and depends on the pathology including systemic and local causes.

Pharmacological treatment like aromatase inhibitors, SERMs, and hCG injections are prescribed for males with testosterone deficiency. Gonadotropins are recommended for males with hypogonadotropic hypogonadism with low levels of LH and FSH. For primary testicular failure, microsurgical procedures for sperm aspiration and extraction are preferred. Novel technologies such as stem cell implants for spermatogenesis and its maintenance are under research to provide hope to patients with testicular failure. Idiopathic male infertility is not benefitted by pharmacological therapy but gonadotropins may be offered to improve pregnancy rates.[9]

■ CONCLUSION

Male infertility evaluation requires a combination of detail history, physical examination, semen analysis, hormonal profile, and imaging and is advised when required. Genetic testing and testicular biopsy requires definite recommendation. Newer research into evaluation of these genetic, genomic, epigenetic, metabolomic defects is suggested for better understanding of male infertility.

REFERENCES

1. World Health Organization. WHO Laboratory Manual for the Examination and Processing of Human Semen, 5 edition. Geneva, Switzerland: WHO Press. 2010. p. 287.
2. Practice Committee of the American Society for Reproductive Medicine. Definitions of infertility and recurrent pregnancy loss: a committee opinion. Fertil Steril. 2020; 113:533-5.
3. Thonneau P, Marchand S, Tallec A, et al. Incidence and main causes of infertility in a resident population (1,850,000) of three French regions (1988–1989). Hum Reprod. 1991;6:811.
4. Rowe T. Fertility and a woman's age. J Reprod Med. 2006;51:157.
5. Dimitriadis F, Adonakis G, Kaponis A, Mamoulakis C, Takenaka A, et al. Pre-testicular, testicular, and post-testicular causes of male infertility. In: Simoni M, Huhtaniemi I (Eds). Endocrinology of the Testis and Male Reproduction. Cham: Springer; 2017. p1364.
6. Guzick DS, Overstreet JW, Factor-Litvak P, et al. Sperm morphology, motility, and concentration in fertile and infertile men. N Engl J Med. 2001; 345:1388.
7. Practice Committee of the American Society for Reproductive Medicine. Diagnostic evaluation of the infertile male: a committee opinion. Fertil Steril. 2015;103:e18.
8. Oliva A and Multigner L. Chronic epididymitis and grade III varicocele and their associations with semen characteristics in men consulting for couple infertility. Asian J Androl. 2018;20:360.
9. Schlegel PN, Sigman M, Collura B, De Jonge CJ, Eisenberg ML, Lamb DJ, Mulhall JP, Niederberger C, Sandlow JI, Sokol RZ, Spandorfer SD, Tanrikut C, Treadwell JR, Oristaglio JT, Zini A. Diagnosis and treatment of infertility in men: AUA/ASRM Guideline Part I. J Urol. 2021;205(1):36-43. doi: 10.1097/JU.0000000000001521. Epub 2020 Dec 9. PMID: 33295257.
10. Behre HM, Bergmann M, Simoni M, et al. Primary testicular failure. [updated 2015 Aug 30]. South Dartmouth, MA: MDText.com, Inc., 2000.
11. Chillon M, Casals T, Mercier B, et al. Mutations in the cystic fibrosis gene in patients with congenital absence of the vas deferens. N Engl J Med. 1995;332:1475.
12. Yu J, Chen Z, Ni Y, et al. CFTR mutations in men with congenital bilateral absence of the vas deferens (CBAVD): a systemic review and meta-analysis. Hum Reprod. 2012;27:25-35.
13. Aitken RJ, Sutton M, Warner P, Richardson DW. Relationship between the movement characteristics of human spermatozoa and their ability to penetrate cervical mucus and zona-free hamster oocytes. J Reprod Fertil. 1985;73:441-9.
14. Mandal M, Saha S, Ghosh AK, Majumder GC. Identification and characterization of a sperm motility promoting glycoprotein from buffalo blood serum. J Cell Physiol. 2006;209:353-62.
15. Dey S, Roy D, Majumder GC, Bhattacharyya D. Extracellular regulation of sperm transmembrane adenylyl cyclase by a forward motility stimulating protein. PLoS One. 2014;9:e110669.
16. Brahem S, Jellad S, Ibala S, Saad A, Mehdi M. DNA fragmentation status in patients with necrozoospermia. Syst Biol Reprod Med. 2012;58(6):319-23.
17. McMahon CG. Disorders of male orgasm and ejaculation. In: Wein AJ, Kavoussi LR, Partin AW, et al (Eds). Campbell-Walsh Urology. Philadelphia: Elsevier, 2016;692-708.
18. Ammar T, Sidhu PS, Wilkins CJ. Male infertility: the role of imaging in diagnosis and management. Br J Radiol. 2012;85(special_issue_1):59-68.
19. Brugh VM, III, Matschke HM, Lipshultz LI. Male factor infertility. Endocrinol Metab Clin North Am. 2003;32(3):689-707.
20. Jarow JP, Espeland MA, Lipshultz LI. Evaluation of the azoospermic patient. J Urol. 1989;142(1):62-5. doi: 10.1016/S0022-5347(17)38662-7.

CHAPTER 3

The Environment and Infertility

Jaya Sharma, Jaideep Malhotra, Divya Yadav

■ INTRODUCTION

Reproductive health is an important part of couple's social and mental wellbeing. We talk lot about detox water and diet and organic food but we are unaware of toxic environment. Humans in their reproductive age are being exposed to small amounts of potentially toxic materials such as lead, mercury and polychlorinated biphenyls (PCBs).

Periconceptional period in human depicts five stages of reproductive development: Gametogenesis, fertilization, embryogenesis, implantation and placentation. A compromised egg or sperm can alter the trajectory of development. A less than optimal environment can predispose an individual to many diseases in adulthood like heart disease, diabetes, obesity and stroke. Our occupation, living style, food habits are major marker of exposure. Over last decade studies in animals and human have shown many such co-relations. Factors thought to affect human fertility are the physical environment, behavioral patterns, socioeconomic factors and environmental contaminants.[1] Chemicals found in our environment have a negative effect on reproductive health and fetal development. More than 85000 synthetic chemicals are being produced and many new are being added per year. Any insult by mimicking or blocking the normal pathway by any harmful agent in environment either food, water or soil will change the expected pathway resulting in various complications. The main routes of exposure to these chemicals is the process of contaminated food and water or through dermal contact or inhalation.[2,3] These agents are knows as Endocrine-disrupting chemicals (EDC). Endocrine disrupting chemical (EDCs) are defined by the Environmental Protection Agency (EPA) as: "Exogenous agents that interferes with the synthesis, secretion, transport, metabolism, binding action, or elimination natural blood-borne hormones that are present in the body and responsible for homeostasis, reproduction and development process."[5]

What we need to understand are:
1. What are the environmental and genetic factors determine the optimum function of egg and sperm?[8]
2. Critical biological events and pathways in periconceptional period that promote or hamper the developmental potential of oocyte and embryo affecting health and functional capacity in later life.
3. Role of environmental conditions, genes, maternal disorders that influence optimum growth of embryo and fetus.
4. Role of male and female factors for infertility.
5. How does the immune response modulated by stress, nutrition, infection, inflammation, metabolic status, resource?

EFFECTS OF EDCs (FIG.1)

Endocrine disrupters are ubiquitous in the environment. Ingestion, inhalation and dermal absorption are the main routes of daily exposure. They cause direct damage to cell membrane and intracellular components.[9]

1. *Mimicking, stimulating, and antagonizing the action of hormones:* They can accumulate in tissues for an extremely long time and experience a conjugation-deconjugation cycling. Thus, their excretion in body is delayed. Some EDCs may accumulate in reproductive organs and act as an endocrine disruptor owing to its structural similarity to hormones. For example, bisphenol acetate (BPA) has a mixed agonist-antagonist to affect estrogens and other steroid hormones. BPA could exert its impact at a very low dose. For example, BPA had estrogenic effects at 2 μg/kg.
2. It causes incomplete development and repair of DNA during fetal development.
3. It changes the microenvironment of seminal plasma, resulting in lower sperm count and motility thereby reducing fertility.
4. Changes follicular microenvironment thereby affecting the number of oocyte retrieved, recovered, and fertilized, cleavage rates and pregnancy rate.
5. Changes amniotic sac environment causing developmental anomalies, pregnancy losses and restricted growth. Fetuses are more vulnerable to the adverse effects of endocrine disrupters. This is because they neither have a gut flora, nor liver to metabolize and also not able to defecate or get rid of toxins through urination. They easily accumulate heavy metals such as mercury which enters human food chain.
6. *Effect on hypothalamus:* It may cause developmental and/or functional defects of the hypothalamic system, which could result in inability to achieve the reproductive capacity at puberty and maintain it during adulthood.[6] It was confirmed that irreversible alteration in hypothalamic-pituitary-gonadal axis caused by exposure to 500 μg/kg/day BPA in rats can lead to anovulation and infertility.[6]
7. *BPA and ovary:* BPA and other EDs have various effects on the ovary like follicle loss, lower antral follicle counts, decreased oocyte survival, and even significant loss of primordial follicles by reducing ovarian follicular reserves in F3 generation females. Studies have suggested a possible role of BPA in PCOS etiopathogenesis. BPA has also been shown to increase testosterone (T) concentration by stimulating ovaries to produce T [50] and inhibiting T-hydroxylase activity.[5]
8. *Effects seminal plasma microenvironment*: Seminal plasma acts as chemical concentrator, increasing the level of various environmental toxicants. Men having higher pesticide levels in blood and semen have lower sperm counts and motility.[2]
9. *Effect on Fallopian tubes*: Studies on mice suggested that, BPA causes progressive proliferative lesions (PPL) in Fallopian tubes.[7]
10. *Effects on uterus animal* studies have demonstrated that prenatal exposure of mice to BPA could elicit atypical hyperplasia and stromal polyps of the uterus, endometriosis-like lesions and also resulted in impaired receptivity,

18   The Environment and Infertility

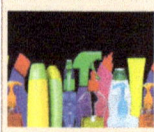
Phthalates
- In plastic toys, shampoo, personal care products, varnishes
- *Effects*: Delayes conception, fetal loss, affects semen quality, ↑anogenital distance

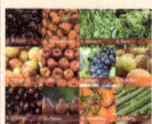
Pesticides
- DDE (Dicholorodiphenyldichloroethylene), DDT (Dicholorodiphenyltrichloronethane), organochlorides found in fruits vegetables, fruits and, soaps
- *Effects*: ↓fecundity, ↓success of IVF, ↓semen quality, ↑preterm birth, ↑SGA, endometriosis, hormonal changes in male

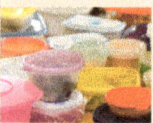
Bisphenols
- Water bottles and plastic food containers
- *Effects*: Oocyte abnormalities, recurrent abortions, poor semen quality

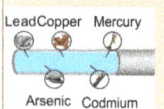
Heavy metals
- Found in paint, pipes, thermometer, farmed fish
- *Effects*: ↓semen quality, ↓fertility, ↑abortion, ↓IQ in offspring

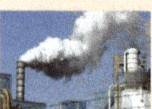
Dioxins
- Industries, fires, fatty meats, fish and dairy products
- *Effects*: ↑endometriosis, birth defects, alters sex ratio

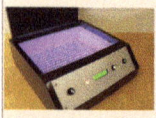
Polychlorinated biphenyl (PCB)
- Found in cutting oils, lubricants, insulators, fish
- *Effects*: ↓response to ovulation induction, ↓sperm quality, ↑endometriosis

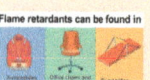
Polybrominated diphenyl ether (PBDE)
- Matteresses, furniture, electronic devices, TV, computers
- *Effects*: Reproductive developemental disruption

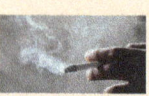
Cigarette smoke
- Active and passive smoking
- *Effects*: ↓fertility, ↑miscarrige, ↓semen quality

Fig. 1: EDCs and their effects

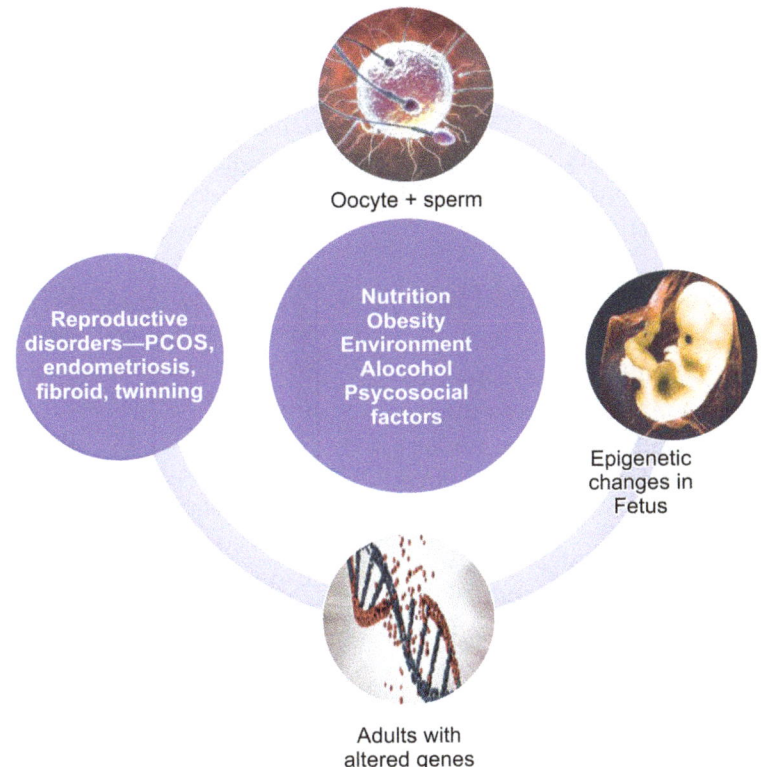

Fig. 2: Effects of external factors

which is important for successful embryo implantation.
- *Physical factors:* Heat exposure to male and noise exposure to female were associated with infertility (Rachootin and Olsen, 1983) **(Fig. 2)**.
- *Psychosocial factors:* Ineffective copulation, different work shifts, work pressure, depression and anxiety are associated with low fecundity.[4] (Jerrell et al., 1993a)
Therefore psychological counseling of couple is important part of treatment.
- Chemical factors having negative impact on Reproductive potential are:
  - Occupational—welding, solvents, agriculture
  - Lifestyle—Smoking, caffeine, alcohol, Mercury-containing fish consumption
  - Others—Air, water and food, electromagnetic radiation and sedentary life
  - Illicit drugs like anabolic steroids
- Female and male weight disorders are linked with fertility outcome by affecting internal hormonal environment thereby reducing ART outcomes, poor pregnancy outcome, increased rate of congenital abnormalities.
- Dietary factors improvising reproduction are the presence of vitamin A, D, iodine, antioxidants rich fruits, vegetables.
- Air pollutants causing infertility

Active or passive smoking causes reduced fecundity in females. Higher rate of spontaneous abortion, still birth, infant mortality and ectopic pregnancy are seen in female's exposure of smoke and other air pollutants. Smoking and other air-induced chemicals also effects male fertility by reducing sperm count, motility, number and density. Closer the women lives near high ways or busy road, higher is the rate of infertility. Air pollutants with biggest impact in this are PM10 and total suspended particulates of SO_2, CO and NOx.[10]

■ PRECONCEPTION PREPARATION

With the available knowledge of environmental factors for infertility, all the clinicians should have a program to assess adverse genetic and lifestyle influence on reproduction and an interventional protocol to reduce their detrimental effects.

Action plan may be in simple steps (**Fig. 3**):
1. Giving general reproductive education for example 'Read labels' while buying edibles.
2. Modification of diet to optimize periconceptional environment.
3. Making weight loss programs.
4. Smoking cessation interventions.
5. Eliminating inappropriate alcohol and drugs.
6. Taking folic acid and antioxidants.
7. Promotion of vaccination like rubella, varicella zoster, herpes before planning conception.
8. Occupational modifications such as a safe workplace, correction of circadian rhythms, avoiding prolonged and heavy workload.
9. Women of child-bearing age should avoid fish that are likely to contain high levels of methyl mercury like sword fish, tile fish, King Mackerel.
10. 'Go organic'. Locally available food usage should be encouraged as, the more distance food travels, the more it is exposed to chemicals.
11. Chemicals should be avoided as far as possible but they are ubiquitous in cosmetics, water, canned food, perfumes, air fresheners and household cleaners. Age old cleansers made by lemon juice and vinegars and essential oils as fresheners can be used.
12. BPA-free bottles should be used for drinking water. Metal and glass bottles to be preferred.
13. Microwaving in plastics should be avoided as much as possible or should be done in *microwave safe plastic*.

Awareness	• Doctor–Patient awareness campaigns
Interviews	• Individual and couple interview regarding lifestyle
Planning	• Reproductive health pathway planning
Advice	• Reproductive health life script
Information	• Reproductive health information sheet
Resources	• Provision of lifestyle resources

Fig. 3: Steps to reduce the effects of external agents on fertility.

■ CONCLUSION

Our health is directly proportional to environmental health and human activities are inversely proportional to environmental health for our good ART results, we need good physical, chemical and psychosocial environment for both male and female partners.

Understanding the various factors that cause oxidative stress in our species and controlling levels of exposure through the imposition of appropriate regulatory frameworks and adoption of relevant protective behavior is very important to reduce harmful effects on human fertility.

Translation of subfertility across generations is one of the most interesting and concerning concepts to arise out of reproductive environmental health research.

Patients should be asked where they live and where they lived, where they work, what they eat, how much fish they consume. Exposure history of couple and their parents to plastic, heavy metal, pesticides and industrial solvents.

In the end, scientific communities at large remain unimpressed with the impact of EDCs. There is much more work needed. Community partnership and support are key.

Some simple habits to limit exposure—Go organic, Read labels, Avoid chemicals, Drink filtered water, Do not microwave in plastic or unmarked containers.

Further studies are needed to confirm whether an environmental relevant dose in accordance with the human natural exposure may cause adverse effects.

■ REFERENCES

1. Younglai V, et al. Environmental and occupational factors affecting fertility and IVF success. Human Reproduction Update. 2005;11 (1);43-57.
2. David K Gardner, et al. Textbook of Assisted Reproductive Techniques.
3. Rachootin and Olsen, 1983
4. Jerrell et al., 1993a
5. Colborn T, Vom Saal FS, Soto AM. Developmental effects of endocrine-disrupting chemicals in wildlife and humans. Environ Health Perspect. 1993;101:378-84.
6. Huo X, Chen D, He Y, Zhu W, Zhou W, Zhang J. Bisphenol-A and female infertility: a possible role of gene-environment interactions International Journal of Environmental Research and Public Health. 2015;12(9):11101-16.
7. Pizzorno J. Environmental Toxins and Infertility. Integr Med (Encinitas). 2018;17(2):8-11. PMID: 30962779; PMCID: PMC6396757.
8. http://www.update.com/contents/occupational and -environmental-risks-to-reproduction-in-females.
9. Brevini TA, Zanetto SB, Cillo F. Effects of endocrine disruptors on developmental and reproductive functions. Curr Drug Targets Immune Endocr Metabol Disord. 2005;5:1-10.
10. Sutton P, Woodruff TJ, Perron J, et al. Toxic environmental chemicals: The role of reproduction – in – females.

CHAPTER 4

Genetics and Infertility

Ruchika Garg, Rekha Rani

■ INTRODUCTION

The search for 'hidden' genetic factors with potential clinical application was largely unsuccessful in identifying recurrent genetic factors. Numerous genetic studies in animal models have identified thousands of genes that are essential for mammalian reproduction. Only less than 200 of these genes shows strong association with human infertility.

In humans, the gonadal development in females and males is identical within first four weeks after conception.

■ MALE INFERTILITY

About 40% of primary testicular failure, the etiology remains unknown and a portion of them is likely to be caused by not yet identified genetic anomalies.

Screening for Y-chromosome-linked gr/gr deletion in those populations for which consistent data with risk estimate are available and Klinefelter's syndrome account for 10–20% of cases of severe spermatogenic failure. 47,XYY males frequently have oligozoospermia or azoospermia but majority are fertile, with normal semen parameters.

Genetic Polymorphisms

Multiple genes are involved but the problem is we only study single genes.

Diagnostic Tests

Single nucleotide polymorphisms and comparative genomic hybridization arrays, concerning deletions) in men with impaired spermatogenesis.

Next generation sequencing (NGS) mutations in several hundred genes can potentially lead to infertility and only a small fraction of cases are attributed by it. System biology, which allows revealing possible gene interactions and common biological pathways, will provide an informative tool for NGS data interpretation.

■ FEMALE INFERTILITY

Defects in Oogenesis

It involves interaction between the oocyte and somatic cells surrounding it, including the interplay of multiple transcriptional regulators.

Embryo development is initially regulated by maternal transcripts that are synthetized and stored in the cytoplasm during oocyte maturation. The euploid maternal genome and the cytoplasmic components are essential for normal embryonic development. Other pathologies, such as disruption of reproductive tract development, endometriosis, uterine fibroids, polycystic ovary syndrome, or autoimmune factors, may have a negative impact on implantation and pregnancy, leading to infertility or recurrent pregnancy loss.

Whole exome and genome sequencing to families with infertility, have led to unbiased approaches and discovered new genes and novel variants involved in human infertility.

Genetics and PCOS

Genomic changes in the *FSHR and other* genes along with noncoding RNAs have been proposed to disturb balance between LH and FSH hormonal stimulation of the thecal and granulosa cells, leading to excessive male hormone and low estradiol concentration in follicle.

Chromosome Segregation Error

X-Chromosome and Female Infertility

In the normal ovary, the primordial germ cells carry two X-chromosomes, one of which is initially inactivated similarly to any other somatic cell. Importantly, the second X-chromosome is reactivated prior to meiosis as the presence of two transcriptionally active X-chromosomes is essential for oogenesis. In females, both X-chromosomes must be active during meiosis to pair efficiently like autosome homologues. Moreover, ~20% of X-linked genes escape inactivation and continue to be expressed from the inactive X-chromosome, maintaining the dosage of female-specific transcripts in surrounding somatic cells.

Monosomy X (Turner syndrome), cytogenetically visible deletions and duplications, and balanced and unbalanced X-autosome rearrangements are associated with an accelerated loss of primordial oocytes during female fetal development, leading to streak gonads accounting for 10% of cases of POI. However, some studies suggest the presence of a surveillance mechanism that may detect and eliminate cells with unpaired or unsynapsed chromatin, such as cells with monosomy X.

Accelerated germ cell depletion by inadequate signaling from surrounding somatic granulosa cells that also carry a single X-chromosome.

Premature Ovarian Failure (POI)

It is characterized by primary or secondary amenorrhea, infertility, decreased estrogen production, elevated gonadotropins (follicle-stimulating hormone and luteinizing hormone).

Failure in either dosage of X-linked genes or the X-chromosome structural integrity can lead to POI. Rossetti et al. found oligogenic nature of POI. Only few X-linked genes have been implicated in ovarian function. *BMP15* located on the human X-chromosome and have been linked with ovarian development and POI.

Beside POI, X-chromosome abnormalities such as deletions, duplications, inversions, complex rearrangements, X-autosome translocations, and single-gene sequence variants, carried by at least 5–6% of women, can lead to recurrent fetal losses.

In females, X-chromosome abnormalities may result in early embryonic or fetal lethality, particularly of male conceptuses.

X-linked genes lead to specific phenotype in humans, pathogenic variants in X-linked genes, such as *BCOR, EBP, FLNA, HCCS, IKBKG, MECP2, OFD1, OTC*, and *REP1*, are presumed to be male-lethal.

Germline mosaicism can lead to infertility and recurrent miscarriages with X-linked or autosomal dominant lethal alteration like pathogenic variants of male-lethal genes *IKBKG, FLNA*, and *MECP2*. Female fetuses can also be affected by male-lethal X-linked disorders in cases of skewed X-chromosome inactivation.

About 15% of individuals with XY gonadal dysgenesis have deletions or pathogenic sequence variants affecting the *SRY* gene on the Y-chromosome.

XY Gonadal Dysgenesis

Y-chromosome structural alterations, mosaicism for a cell line with monosomy X, heterozygous deletions, and sequence variants in the *NR5A1* gene, duplications in the Xp21 region involving *NR0B1*, *WNT4* gene duplications, and deletions.

Mitochondrial dysfunction can lead to defects in oocyte maturation, impaired spindle assembly and chromosome mis-segregation, poor pre-implantation development, and implantation failure.

XX Gonadal Dysgenesis

Ovarian development is orchestrated by several transcription factors, including *SOHLH1*, *SOHLH2*, *NOBOX*, etc., mitotic proliferation of XX primordial germ cells, their progression into meiosis, and the formation of primordial follicles.

Defects in Folliculogenesis

Multiple oocyte-specific transcription factors, like *FIGLA*, control follicular development. In mice, these genes are autosomal recessive and this is likely to be true in humans, but further studies only will be able to tell whether heterozygous variants in these genes can cause pathology.

DNA Repair Genes

Defects in repairing chromosomal ends activates cell apoptosis, leading to depletion of germ cells and loss of ovarian reserves.

■ CONCLUSION

Mouse studies found that *Sohlh1* and *Sohlh2* affect differentiation of both male and female gametes, while *Nobox*, *Lhx8*, and *Figla* are gamete-specific genes which regulate only oogenesis, and not male germ cell differentiation. Orthologues of such mouse genes are present in our genome. Structural X-chromosome abnormalities, rather than gene-specific abnormalities, may be the major reason for germ cell loss.

These recent genome-wide association studies have been able to throw light on only a small number of human infertility genes, and more discoveries are expected in the near future.

■ BIBLIOGRAPHY

1. Aston KI. Genetic susceptibility to male infertility: news from genome-wide association studies. Andrology. 2014; 2(3):315-21. doi: 10.1111/j.2047-2927. 2014.00188.x. Epub 2014 Feb 19. PMID: 24574159.
2. Marongiu M, Crisponi L, Uda M, Pelosi E. Editorial: Female Infertility: Genetics of Reproductive Ageing, Menopause and Primary Ovarian Insufficiency. Front Genet. 2022;13:839758. doi: 10.3389/fgene. 2022.839758.
3. Yatsenko SA, Rajkovic A. Genetics of human female infertility. Biol Reprod. 2019;101(3):549-66. doi: 10.1093/biolre/ioz084. PMID: 31077289; PMCID: PMC8127036.
4. Zorrilla M, Yatsenko AN. The genetics of infertility: current status of the field. Curr Genet Med Rep. 2013;247-60. https://doi.org/10.1007/s40142-013-0027-1.

CHAPTER 5

Nutrition and Infertility

Sufia Naseem, Shaheen Anjum

■ INTRODUCTION

Infertility is the failure to establish a clinical pregnancy after a year of regular, unprotected sexual contact. It is characterized by an impairment of a person's capacity to reproduce as an individual or with his/her partner.[1] It is estimated that it affects roughly 15% of reproductive-aged couples attempting pregnancy worldwide.[2]

Studies suggest that approximately one in every eight couple experiences difficulty becoming pregnant. Female infertility contributes to only 35% of overall infertility cases; 20% of cases are related to both women and men; 30% involve problems only on the part of men; and 15% of infertility cases remain unexplained.[3,4] Nutrition and other environmental factors influence women's reproductive health and the outcomes of assisted reproductive technologies (ART).

Evidence suggests that nutrition can play an essential role in altering fertility-related results. Panth et al.[5] As a matter of fact, research suggests that a diet high in processed carbohydrates, trans fats, and added sugars may have a detrimental effect on fertility. In contrast, a diet focused on Mediterranean dietary patterns, i.e., high in dietary fiber, omega-3 fatty acids, plant-based protein, vitamins, and minerals, has a beneficial effect on female fertility.[6] An unhealthy diet may alter microbiota composition, and it is critical to determine whether the frequency of infertility correlates with gut microbiota composition. There is not enough proof that every woman trying to get pregnant should cut gluten out of her diet if she does not have celiac disease. Also, there is no information about how drinking alcohol might hurt a woman's fertility, and drinking the right amount of caffeine does not seemingly affect fertility.[7,8] On the other hand, phytoestrogens presumably positively influence female fertility. There is still a lot to unearth how diet affects female fertility, although genomic, epigenetic, and microbial pathways may be involved. Therefore, it is the need of the hour to uncover the intricate impact of nutritional factors on infertility in particular and this study has focused on the effects of dietary variables on female fertility. The aim of this chapter is to sum up the nutritional aspects related to infertility.

There is a lot of evidence that healthy eating habits before pregnancy are good for fertility in both men and women of childbearing age. The US Dietary Guidelines, recommend a high intake of vegetables, fruits, fish, whole grains and monounsaturated or polyunsaturated oils,[9] and have been linked to enhanced female fertility and better semen quality.[10]

In the Nurses' Health Study (NHS) II, participants who mostly consumed a "fertility diet", which included full-fat dairy products, iron, and monounsaturated fats, had a 27% lower risk of infertility due to other causes and a 66% lower risk of infertility due to ovulatory disorders.

In another research of college-educated women in Spain, those who adhered to a Mediterranean-style diet, which also included high intakes of vegetables, seafood, and polyunsaturated fats, were 44% less likely to seek medical assistance for getting pregnant.[11]

In Greece, non-obese women found that the Mediterranean diet had similar effects on achieving clinical pregnancy and live birth, but only for those below 35 years of age.[12] Additionally, research shows that eating a balanced diet that includes the foods mentioned above enhances indicators of semen quality such as morphology, motility, and concentration.[13] A healthy diet is vital for a normal reproductive process. In developing countries, most infertile men and women are undernourished. At the same time, in well-developed and western societies, infertility is linked to overeating, eating fast food, eating diets high in calories, and being overweight. A more profound understanding of the molecular processes that are out of order in malnourished people can help us find solutions for re-establishing normal reproductive functioning.

It is especially true for women, where improper nutrition may have a long-lasting impact on oocyte maturation.

■ MALNUTRITION

Deficient food intake and a general lack of nutrients result in loss of both body weight and physical performance, delayed puberty, lengthening of the post-partum interval to conception, lower gonadotropin secretion levels with alterations of the physiological ovarian cyclicity, and increased infertility.

Poor protein, micro- and macro-mineral, and vitamin intake are linked to decreased reproductive performance, as altered energy balance is directly related to decreased ovulatory maturation in women.[14] Thus, inadequate nutrition is closely linked to female reproductive outcomes. The finding that both bulimia nervosa and anorexia, affecting 5% of women of childbearing age, are indisputable causes of amenorrhea, infertility, and miscarriages supports the view.[15]

Overweight and Obesity

The prevalence of overweight or obesity among patients seeking infertility treatment might range from 20 to 25% during the woman's reproductive years. According to the WHO, 9% to 25% of women in industrialized nations are obese. These women are more likely to give birth to fat children, especially if they have gestational diabetes.

Adipose tissue is responsible for ovulatory abnormalities in predisposed people through insulin resistance (IR), high levels of insulin and androgens, and the anovulation linked with obesity is responsible for a higher incidence of miscarriages and infertility.[16] Alongside conventional ovulation induction techniques, diet and exercise treat anovulation in obese women. Obesity and overweight lengthen the gestation period in patients without ovulatory problems.

Therefore, the modification of lifestyle habits and unhealthy behaviors by appropriate assistance or specific management, such as folic acid supplementation, must be provided to females attempting to conceive.[17]

■ HEALTHY NUTRITION FOR A HEALTHY OVULATION

Contrary to the harmful impact of body weight, nutrition significantly improves reproductive efficiency in both men and women. The link between nutrition and fertility appears crucial for reproductive success. The association between ovulatory problems and metabolic diseases such as diabetes and galactosemia implies that dietary factors may be a cause of some types of infertility.[18]

Female and male pre-conceptional nutritional status affects fertility and perinatal problems, according to a 2006 study that included 12,579 participants from the Southampton Women's Survey.[19,20] A prospective observational study found a linear relationship between red blood cell folate and blood and follicular fluid vitamin B6 levels and a diet high in fish, legumes, and vegetables and low in carbohydrates, with a 40% increase in the likelihood of pregnancy by IVF intracytoplasmic sperm injection (ICSI).[21] Similarly, women who undergo IVF/ICSI are more likely to succeed if they consume dietary sources of omega-3 fatty acids (FAs), alpha-linolenic acid, and docosahexaenoic acid (DHA).[22]

The following sections summarize the various nutrients and their potential effects on female fertility.

Proteins

The influence of a protein diet on fertility and ovulation is complicated, and how the type or quantity of protein consumed may affect these processes is still unknown. Protein consumption, however, has been linked to the deregulation of steroidogenesis in PCOS-affected women, most likely via lowering hyperinsulinemia. To illustrate the potential link between protein intake and androgen production, Mumford et al. showed that in healthy women, a diet high in protein, especially animal proteins, is strongly associated with lower testosterone levels.[23]

Carbohydrates

The possibility that carbohydrate consumption may impact ovulatory function and general fertility in healthy women is still debatable. In this situation, healthy women with PCOS were seen to have regained ovulatory function and fertility by enhancing glucose homeostasis. Because of this, the effects of carbohydrate intake on glucose metabolism are likely to cause different ovulatory problems.[24]

A higher glycemic load in the diet is linked to higher fasting glucose levels, hyperinsulinemia, and IR, which are then linked to higher free IGF-I and androgen release, leading to endocrine disruption and abnormalities in oocyte maturation.[25]

Lipids

Much research is being done on how lipids affect female fertility. It is hypothesized that dietary fatty acid and cholesterol intakes affect fertility and pregnancy outcomes, most likely by increasing the production of prostaglandins and steroids.[26] However, more information is needed regarding the connection between dietary fat, androgen levels, and ovulation.

Mumford, et al. found that total fat intakes of polyunsaturated fatty acids (PUFA) were not linked to higher testosterone levels in 259 women who had regular periods. Instead, they were linked to higher progesterone levels, making anovulation less likely.[27] So, their results suggest that fatty acids, especially PUFAs, do not play a significant role in making androgens.

However, extensive research is required to determine whether or not changes in androgen synthesis would consistently affect female fertility.

Vitamins and Minerals

Exogenous oligo-elements and vitamins can be obtained from food; hence current clinical practice advises combining dietary supplements with a healthy diet to correct this imbalance, induce OS control, and enhance fertility.[28] Among the many antioxidants currently in use, glutathione is a naturally occurring substance with potent detoxification properties that protects cells from free radical damage by inhibiting their formation.

Ascorbic acid's effects have been extensively documented in the literature, and it has been shown that ascorbic acid ingestion during pregnancy may boost the trophoblastic steroidogenesis that physiologically supports gestation.[29] It has also been noted that the blood ascorbic acid levels were lower in females with numerous spontaneous miscarriages caused by a luteal phase abnormality than in females with better reproductive results.[30]

Antioxidants

Oxidative stress results from an imbalance in the body's defense mechanisms against free radicals (ROS) and their release.[31] Reproductive ability may be impacted by oxidative stress (OS) and the subsequent variance in DNA methylation.

However, despite several studies demonstrating the impact of antioxidant intake on the ability to reproduce, less is known about how they affect menstruation function.[32]

According to a report from the BioCycle Study, there is no link between FSH and sex hormone-binding globulin (SHBG), although there is a significant correlation between oxidative stress and endogenous estradiol (E2).[33]

Despite antioxidants' helpful role in lowering the OS, Showell, et al. found that their improper or excessive use could have some adverse effects.[34] Therefore, more research is required to learn how antioxidants affect the body to enhance reproductive success.

Folates

It is well known that taking 400 g of folic acid every day in the preconceptional period will raise folate levels and lower homocysteine (Hcy) levels in follicular fluid.

Folic acid supplements or multivitamins with folic acid have been linked to a higher quality embryo, a higher chance of getting pregnant, and a lower risk of ovulatory infertility.[35]

However, barely 50% of infertile women use these products correctly throughout the preconception period, despite the fact that over 80% of them respond to folic acid supplementation and that infertile women take it more frequently than fertile women.[36]

Murto, et al. looked at the folate levels of fertile and infertile women in this case. They found that fertile women had a much better folate status than infertile women, and infertile patients were more likely than controls to take folic acid supplements.[37]

Folates are a class of interconvertible coenzymes essential for protein, DNA, and methylation synthesis. A lack of folate may interfere with these chemical interactions, causing Hcy buildup and excess OS.

An epigenetic mechanism called DNA methylation can alter the expression of particular genes without altering the DNA sequence.

Additionally, methylation changes how physically accessible the nucleic acids are to the molecular complexes involved in gene expression, which may modify or suppress the function of the genes.

Numerous molecular processes, including embryonic development, gene transcription, X-chromosome inactivation, genomic imprinting, chromosome stability, and cell division, are all impacted by this process. Thus, independent of the DNA sequence, the information is passed on to the daughter cells.[38]

THE MEDITERRANEAN DIET (MED DIET)

The Mediterranean diet is a nutritious eating plan that was influenced by the 1950s dietary trends of people in Greece, Southern Italy, and Spain. The main parts of this diet are eating a lot of fruits, vegetables, legumes, olive oil, unrefined grains, moderate-to-high amounts of fish, wine, and less meat.

The Mediterranean diet was linked to higher folate and vitamin B_6 levels in the blood and follicular fluid, making it 40% more likely that a woman would get pregnant.[39]

Recent research suggests that preconception diets may affect the success of IVF.

Karayiannis, et al. and his colleagues looked at how the Med Diet affected how well IVF worked for women trying to get pregnant. They found no association between the Med Diet and the results of IVF or the frequency of implantation.[12]

SPECIFIC FOODS AND NUTRIENTS

A critical understanding of the probable mechanisms behind the association between diet and reproductive health may be gained from data on the correlations between specific nutrients and fertility.

Low folate levels are linked to less sporadic anovulation and neural tube abnormalities in babies.[40] In a three-month, double-blind, randomized controlled trial, 26% of women with low fertility who took 400 mg/day of folic acid got pregnant, compared to 10% of those who took a placebo.[41]

According to preliminary studies, red meat may negatively impact fertility. It has been discovered that red meat's high saturated fat content is associated with men's decreased semen concentration.[42] The full-fat dairy products showed a lower risk of ovulatory infertility, while low-fat dairy products (such as skim, 1%, and 2% milk, yogurt, or cottage cheese) were linked to a higher risk.

CONCLUSION

Eating well can help medical treatments such as IVF and fertility treatments work better. Incorporating healthy eating, movement, and exercise into a healthy lifestyle will assist in obtaining an ideal weight. Whole grains help stabilize blood sugar to prevent hormonal fluctuations that can disrupt fertility. Ingestion of whole grains is linked to a higher chance of having a live birth. Avoiding refined carbohydrates (white bread, pasta, sugary cereals, soda, fruit juices, and cookies) and consuming more whole grains (whole grain bread, cereals, pasta, whole fruits, and beans) should be considered. The focus should be on plant-forward and choline-rich protein sources, including beans, lentils, soy, nuts, seeds, and quinoa. Foods with trans fats should be avoided, including hydrogenated oils, packaged snacks, baked goods, fried foods, shortening, and margarine. Choose heart-healthy unsaturated fats such as avocados, olive oil, nuts (almonds and walnuts), seeds, and fatty fish, including omega-3-rich fish (think salmon), two times per week. Eating seafood before and during pregnancy is recommended twice a week. Iron has also been shown to lower the risk of infertility, so taking a multivitamin with iron or consuming greater amounts of non-heme iron food sources may help. Eating foods high in antioxidants can help ART couples have more live births, especially men. Vitamin C, found in citrus fruits and sunflower seeds, and beta-carotene, found in orange foods such as sweet potatoes and carrots, are good antioxidants.[43]

REFERENCES

1. Thoma ME, McLain AC, Louis JF, King RB, Trumble AC, Sundaram R, et al. Prevalence of infertility in the United States as estimated by the current duration approach and a traditional constructed approach. Fertil Steril. 2013;99:1324-31e1. doi: 10.1016/j.fertnstert.2012.11.037
2. Thurston L, Abbara A, Dhillo WS. Investigation and management of subfertility. J Clin Pathol. 2019;72(9):579-87.
3. Leaver RB. Male infertility: an overview of causes and treatment options. Br J Nurs. 2016;25(18):S35-40.
4. Skoracka K, Ratajczak AE, Rychter AM, Dobrowolska A, Krela-Kaźmierczak I. Female fertility and the nutritional approach: the most essential aspects. Adv Nutr. 2021;12(6):2372-86.
5. Panth N, Gavarkovs A, Tamez M, Mattei J. The influence of diet on fertility and the implications for public health nutrition in the United States. Front Public Health. 2018;6:211.
6. Li K, Huang T, Zheng J, Wu K, Li D. Effect of marine-derived n-3 polyunsaturated fatty acids on C-reactive protein, interleukin 6 and tumor necrosis factor α: a meta-analysis. PLoS One. 2014;9(2):e88103.
7. Dejong K, Olyaei A, Lo JO. Alcohol use in pregnancy. Clin Obstet Gynecol. 2019;62(1):142-55.
8. Chavarro JE, Rich-Edwards JW, Rosner BA, Willett WC. Caffeinated and alcoholic beverage intake in relation to ovulatory disorder infertility. Epidemiology. 2009;20:374-81.
9. US Department of Health and Human Services. US Department of Agriculture. 2015-2020 Dietary Guidelines for Americans. 8th edn. Washington, DC: US Department of Health and Human Services, 2015.
10. Gaskins AJ, Chavarro JE. Diet and fertility: a review. Am J Obstet Gynecol. 2018;218:379-89. doi: 10.1016/j.ajog.2017.08.010.
11. Toledo E, Lopez-del Burgo C, Ruiz-Zambrana A, Donazar M, Navarro-Blasco I, Martinez-Gonzalez MA, et al. Dietary patterns and difficulty conceiving: a nested case-control study. Fertil Steril. 2011; 96:1149-53.
12. Karayiannis D, Kontogianni MD, Mendorou C, Mastrominas M, Yiannakouris N. Adherence to the Mediterranean diet and IVF success rate among non-obese women attempting fertility. Hum Reprod. 2018;33:494-502.
13. Salas-Huetos A, Bullo M, Salas-Salvado J. Dietary patterns, foods and nutrients in male fertility parameters and fecundability: a systematic review of observational studies. Hum Reprod Update. 2017;23:371-89.
14. Jokela M, Elovainio M, Kivimäki M. Lower fertility associated with obesity and underweight: the US National Longitudinal Survey of Youth. Am J Clin Nutr. 2008;88:886-93. doi: 10.1093/ajcn/88.4.886.
15. Group ECW. Nutrition and reproduction in women. Hum Reproduc Update. 2006;12:193-207. doi: 10.1093/humupd/dmk003.
16. WHO. Obesity and Overweight. Geneva, 2013.
17. Bellver J, Ayllon Y, Ferrando M, Melo M, Goyri E, Pellicer A, et al. Female obesity impairs in vitro fertilization outcome without affecting embryo quality. Fertility Steril. 2010;93:447-54. doi: 10.1016/j.fertnstert.2008.12.032.
18. Livshits A, Seidman DS. Fertility issues in women with diabetes. Women's Health. 2009; 5:701-7.
19. Iniguez G, Torrealba IM, Avila A, Cassorla F, Codner E. Adiponectin serum levels and their relationships to androgen concentrations and ovarian volume during puberty in girls with type 1 diabetes mellitus. Hormone Res. 2008;70:112-7.
20. Inskip HM, Godfrey KM, Robinson SM, Law CM, Barker DJ, Cooper C, et al. Cohort profile: the Southampton Women's Survey. Int J Epidemiol. 2006;35:42-8.

21. Vujkovic M, de Vries JH, Lindemans J, Macklon NS, van der Spek PJ, Steegers EA, et al. The preconception Mediterranean dietary pattern in couples undergoing in vitro fertilization/intracytoplasmic sperm injection treatment increases the chance of pregnancy. Fertility Steril. 2010;94:2096-101.
22. Hammiche F, Vujkovic M, Wijburg W, de Vries JH, Macklon NS, Laven JS, et al. Increased preconception omega-3 polyunsaturated fatty acid intake improves embryo morphology. Fertility Steril. 2011;95:1820-3.
23. Mumford SL, Alohali A, Wactawski-Wende J. Dietary protein intake and reproductive hormones and ovulation: the BioCycle study. Fertility Steril. 2015;104:e2.
24. Mioni R, Chiarelli S, Xamin N, Zuliani L, Granzotto M, Mozzanega B, et al. Evidence for the presence of glucose transporter 4 in the endometrium and its regulation in polycystic ovary syndrome patients. J Clin Endocrinol Metabol. 2004;89:4089-96.
25. Chavarro JE, Rich-Edwards JW, Rosner BA, Willett WC. A prospective study of dietary carbohydrate quantity and quality in relation to risk of ovulatory infertility. Eur J Clin Nutr. 2009;63:78-86.
26. Saldeen P, Saldeen T. Women and omega-3 fatty acids. Obstetr Gynecol Survey. 2004;59:722-30; quiz 45–6.
27. Mumford SL, Chavarro JE, Zhang C, Perkins NJ, Sjaarda LA, Pollack AZ, et al. Dietary fat intake and reproductive hormone concentrations and ovulation in regularly menstruating women. Am J Clin Nutr. 2016;103:868-77.
28. Cornet D, Amar E, Cohen M, Ménézo Y. Clinical evidence for the importance of 1-carbon cycle support in subfertile couples. Austin J Reprod Med Infertil. 2015;2:1011. Available online at: https://www.researchgate.net/profile/Yves_Menezo/publication/278381279_Austin_Journal_of_Reproductive_Medicine_Infertility/links/59dce0d30f7e9bdd752dd6a5/Austin-Journal-ofReproductive-Medicine-Infertility.pdf.
29. Wu X, Iguchi T, Itoh N, Okamoto K, Takagi T, Tanaka K, et al. Ascorbic acid transported by sodium-dependent vitamin C transporter 2 stimulates steroidogenesis in human choriocarcinoma cells. Endocrinology. 2008;149:73-83.
30. Vural P, Akgul C, Yildirim A, Canbaz M. Antioxidant defence in recurrent abortion. Clin Chim Acta Int J Clin Chem. 2000;295:169-77.
31. Ferroni P, Barbanti P, Della-Morte D, Palmirotta R, Jirillo E, Guadagni F. Redox mechanisms in migraine: novel therapeutics and dietary interventions. Antioxidants Redox Signal. 2018;28:1144-83.
32. Mayne ST, Wright ME, Cartmel B. Assessment of antioxidant nutrient intake and status for epidemiologic research. J Nutr. 2004;134:3199S-200S.
33. Schisterman EF, Gaskins AJ, Mumford SL, Browne RW, Yeung E, Trevisan M, et al. Influence of endogenous reproductive hormones on F2-isoprostane levels in premenopausal women: the BioCycle Study. Am J Epidemiol. 2010;172:430-9.
34. Showell MG, Brown J, Clarke J, Hart RJ. Antioxidants for female subfertility. Cochr Database Syst Rev. (2013);8:CD007807.
35. Chavarro JE, Rich-Edwards JW, Rosner BA, Willett WC. Use of multivitamins, intake of B vitamins, and risk of ovulatory infertility. Fertility Steril. 2008;89:668-76.
36. Nouri K, Walch K, Weghofer A, Imhof M, Egarter C, Ott J. The Impact of a standardized oral multinutrient supplementation on embryo quality in in vitro fertilization/intracytoplasmic sperm injection: a prospective randomized trial. Gynecol Obstetr Invest. 2017;82:8-14.
37. Murto T, Skoog Svanberg A, Yngve A, Nilsson TK, Altmae S, Wanggren K, et al. Folic acid supplementation and IVF pregnancy outcome in women with unexplained infertility. Reproduc Biomed Online. 2014;28: 766-72.
38. Sivestris E, Cohen M, Menezo Y. Oxidative stress (OS) and DNA methylation errors in reproduction: a place for a support of the one carbon cycle (1-C cycle) before conception. Womens Health Gynecol. 2016;2:30.

39. Vujkovic M, de Vries JH, Lindemans J, Macklon NS, van der Spek PJ, Steegers EA, et al. The preconception Mediterranean dietary pattern in couples undergoing in vitro fertilization/intracytoplasmic sperm injection treatment increases the chance of pregnancy. Fertility Steril. 2010;94:2096-101.
40. Oostingh EC, Hall J, Koster MPH, Grace B, Jauniaux E, Steegers-Theunissen RPM. The impact of maternal lifestyle factors on periconception outcomes: a systematic review of observational studies. Reproduc Biomed Online. 2019;38:77-94.
41. Klonoff-Cohen H, Natarajan L. The concerns during assisted reproductive technologies (CART) scale and pregnancy outcomes. Fertility Steril. 2004;81:982-8.
42. Miller N, Herzberger EH, Pasternak Y, Klement AH, Shavit T, Yaniv RT, et al. Does stress affect IVF outcomes? A prospective study assessing cortisol levels and stress questionnaires for women undergoing through IVF treatments. Reproduc Biomed Online. 2019; S1472-6483(19):30062-8. doi: 10.1016/j.rbmo.2019.01.012.
43. Sivestris E, Cohen M, Menezo Y. Oxidative stress (OS) and DNA methylation errors in reproduction: a place for a support of the one carbon cycle (1-C cycle) before conception. Womens Health Gynecol. 2016;2:30.

CHAPTER 6

Ultrasound Evaluation of Infertility

Maneesha Jain, Narendra Malhotra

Ultrasound (USG) is the most essential imaging tool for diagnosing and treating infertility problems. Transvaginal sonography (TVS) is the modality of choice for assessment of female genital tract and management of infertile females. With the advent of TVS and 3D imaging, there has been a major breakthrough in the infertility field. Ultrasound and Doppler in infertile females is used for these two main purposes:
1. Evaluation of uterine, ovarian and adnexal pathology.
2. Monitoring of stimulated cycle, oocyte retrieval, embryo transfer in the assisted reproductive technology (ART).

All patients with infertility should have baseline TVS scan especially in the early follicular phase. It includes:
1. *Evaluation of the uterus:* Uterus is screened in sagittal and transverse planes. Position, size, mobility, texture of myometrium in terms of thickness, homogeneity, presence of mass, uniformity of the endometrium, endomyometrial junction (EMJ), cervix and cervical canal assessment is done.
2. *Evaluation of ovaries:* Volume, AFC (Antral follicle count) stromal echogenicity and detection of cyst.
3. *Evaluation of tube:* Tubes are usually not seen on a pelvic ultrasound except when hydrosalpinx is there. Apart from this, peritoneal cyst and pelvic adhesions can also be assessed.

EVALUATION OF UTERUS

■ CONGENITAL ANOMALY

Congenital anomalies can be diagnosed by TVS but 3D ultrasound (USG) is recommended because of its high predictive value **(Table 1)**. Bicornuate, Arcuate and subseptate uterus can be differentiated by 3D USG **(Figs 1, 2, 3)**.

The recent European Society of Human Reproduction and Embryology, European society of Gynecological Endoscopy ESHRE-ESGE consensus on the diagnosis of uterine anomaly recommend performing 3D in mid cycle/luteal phase **(Table 2)**.[1]

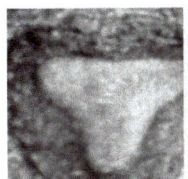 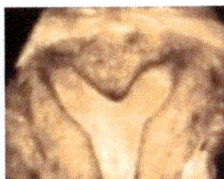 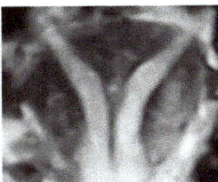 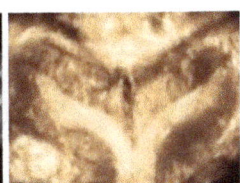 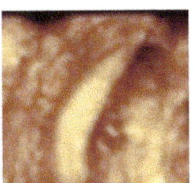

Fig. 1: *Three-dimensional coronal plane of uterus:* Normal uterus, subseptate uterus, septate uterus, bicornuate, unicornuate uterus.

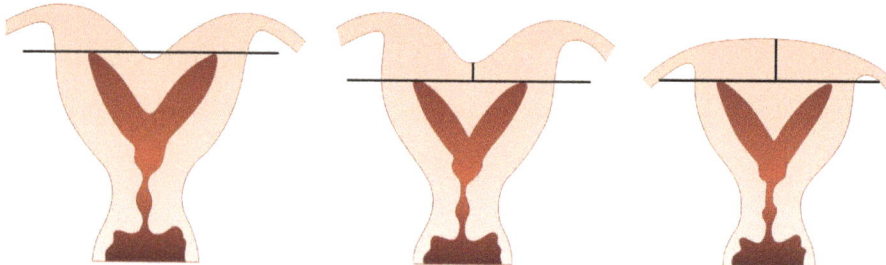

Fig. 2: Bicornuate uterus can be distinguished from septate uterus by using Troiano and McCarthy formula. A line is traced joining both horns of the uterine cavity. If this line crosses the fundus or is ≤5 mm from it, the uterus is considered bicornuate and if it is >5 mm from the fundus, it is considered septate regardless of whether the fundus is dome-shaped or notched.[2]

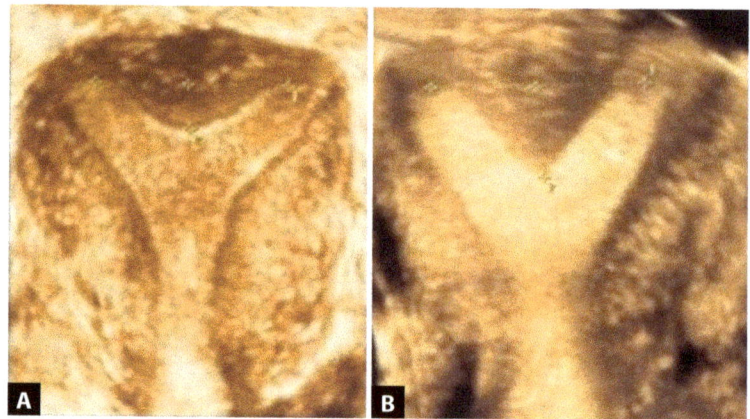

Figs. 3A and B: (A) The fundal indentation appears as obtuse at the central point, <1.5 cm deep in arcuate uterus; (B) Septate uterus is differentiated from arcuate uterus because fundal indentation is acute angle at central point, and >1.5 cm deep.[3,4]

TABLE 1: Three-dimensional ultrasound (3D USG) criteria for classification of congenital uterine anomaly.		
Uterine morphology	**Fundal contour**	**External contour**
Normal	Straight or convex	Uniformly convex with or indentation <10 mm
Arcuate	Concave fundal indentation with central point of indentation at obtuse angle (>90°)	Uniformly convex or with indentation <10 mm
Partial septate	Presence of septum (does not extend to cervix) with central point of septum at an acute angle (<90°)	Uniformly convex or with indentation <10 mm
Complete septate	Presence of septum that completely divides cavity from fundus to cervix	Uniformly convex or with indentation <10 mm
Bicornuate	Two well-formed uterine cornua	Fundal indentation >10 mm dividing the two cornua
Unicornuate uterus	Single well-formed uterine cavity with a single interstitial portion of Fallopian tube and concave fundal contour	Fundal indentation >10 mm dividing the two cornua, if a rudimentary horn is present

TABLE 2: ESHRE/ESGE classification of uterine anomalies.

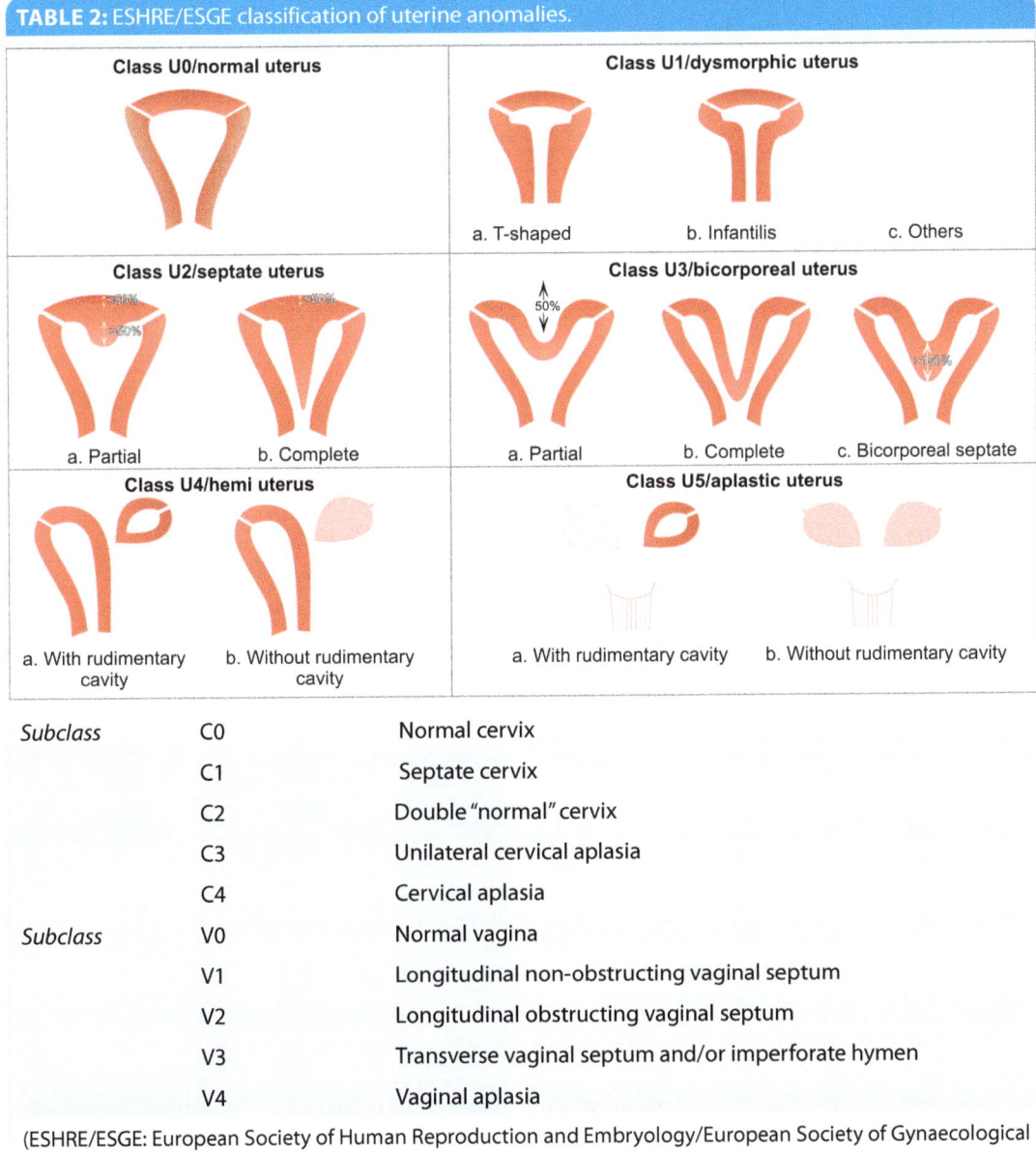

Subclass	C0	Normal cervix
	C1	Septate cervix
	C2	Double "normal" cervix
	C3	Unilateral cervical aplasia
	C4	Cervical aplasia
Subclass	V0	Normal vagina
	V1	Longitudinal non-obstructing vaginal septum
	V2	Longitudinal obstructing vaginal septum
	V3	Transverse vaginal septum and/or imperforate hymen
	V4	Vaginal aplasia

(ESHRE/ESGE: European Society of Human Reproduction and Embryology/European Society of Gynaecological Endoscopy)

MYOMETRIUM

It is normally homogeneously, hypo-echoic with smooth serosa. Myometrial lesions include fibroids, adenomyoma and adenomyosis.

Fibroid

Fibroids are hypo-echoic homogeneous, rounded, solid lesions with well-defined margins.
- These may be calcified.

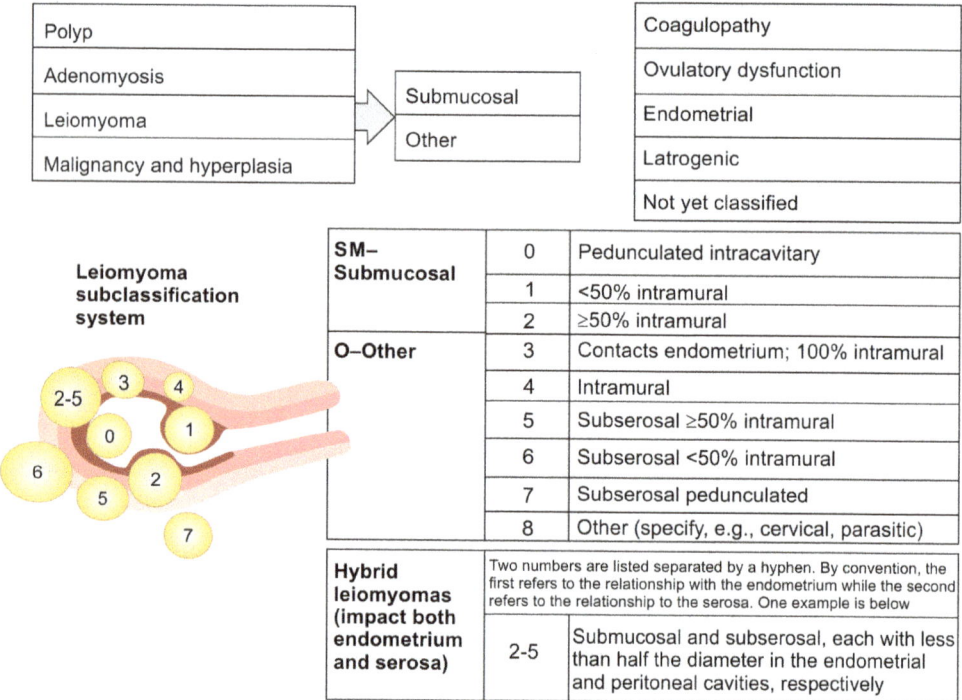

Fig. 4: FIGO classification of fibroid.

- Degeneration may cause heterogeneity in texture.
- Echogenicity increases with increase in vascularity and amount of fibrous tissue.

Fibroids are of importance because:
- Presence of fibroid near endometrium can cause stretching and atrophy of glands along with altered blood flow.
- Distortion of cavity due to submucosal fibroid.
- There is an altered hormonal environment because of fibroid.

Ultrasound plays an important role in assessing the size, invasion, distortion of cavity and is useful in follow-up of patients with medical management **(Fig. 4)**.

Submucosal fibroids are of much importance in infertility:
- *Type 0:* If they are pedunculated and 100% in cavity **(Fig. 5)**

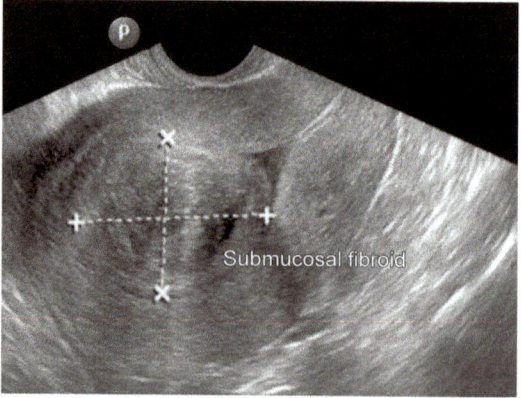

Fig. 5: Submucosal fibroid.

- *Type 1:* If the fibroid is >50% in cavity
- *Type 2:* If fibroid is <50% in cavity
- *Type 0 and 2* can be removed hysteroscopically whereas type 2 needs laparoscopy.

Subserosal and intramural fibroid can be classified as:
- *Type 0:* Pedunculated

- *Type 1:* <50% involvement of outer uterine wall
- *Type 2:* >50% of myometrial wall
- *Type 3:* Fibroid extending from mucosa to serosa.

Adenomyosis (Fig. 6)

- Common in multiparous females.
- It has indistinct margins.
- It is characterized by big, regular heterogeneous uterine mass containing tiny cystic lesions of 2–9 mm. There are alternate vertical hyperechoic and hypoechoic areas in myometrium typically described as 'Swiss-cheese' appearance, 'Rain in forest'.[5]
- Typical speckled appearance hyperechoic and hypoechoic areas known as 'salt and pepper' appearance.[5]
- It can be localized or generalized. Typically characterized by asymmetrical thickening of myometrium.
- Myometrial cysts can be seen. Pressing the uterus can cause pain.
- There is loss of endometrial myometrial junction.

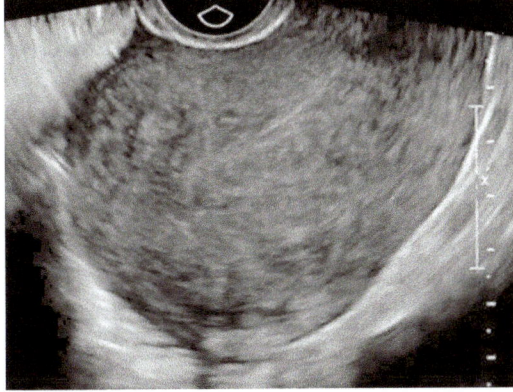

Fig. 6: Sagittal TVS image showing diffuse bulkiness and heterogeneity of myometrium. There is asymmetric thickening of anterior myometrium, pencil thin posterior shadows and obscured border between endometrium and myometrium.

- On color Doppler, affected myometrium shows markedly increased vascularity with vascular clumps. Decreased uterine artery resistance and increased velocity may be seen with large areas of adenomyosis.

More difficult situation is the adenomyoma. This is a localized adenomyosis. When seen in the follicular phase it appears hypo-echoic like a fibroid and if fibroid is degenerated it looks like adenomyoma. But it alters its echogenicity with the phase of the cycle. The main differentiating point between the adenomyoma and the fibroid is the capsular vascularity that is seen in fibroid but is never seen in adenomyoma.

ENDOMETRIUM

Endometrium undergoes changes in accordance with follicular and luteal phase of the ovary during normal menstrual cycles.

Endometrial Thickness

Endometrial thickness is defined as the maximal distance between the echogenic interface of myometrium and endometrium. The Endometrium is thin <5 mm in thickness, post-menses **(Fig. 7A)**. A triple-lined echotexture pattern >11 mm is seen in near ovulatory phase **(Fig. 7B)**. 3D USG provide a better view.

Endometrial Pattern

It is the relative echogenicity of endometrium and myometrium on longitudinal TVS. Gonen and Casper proposed 3 grade system.[6]

Grade A: Entirely homogeneous, hyperechogenic pattern, without a central echogenic line.

Grade B: Isoechogenic pattern, with same echogenicity as surrounding myometrium, without a central echogenic line.

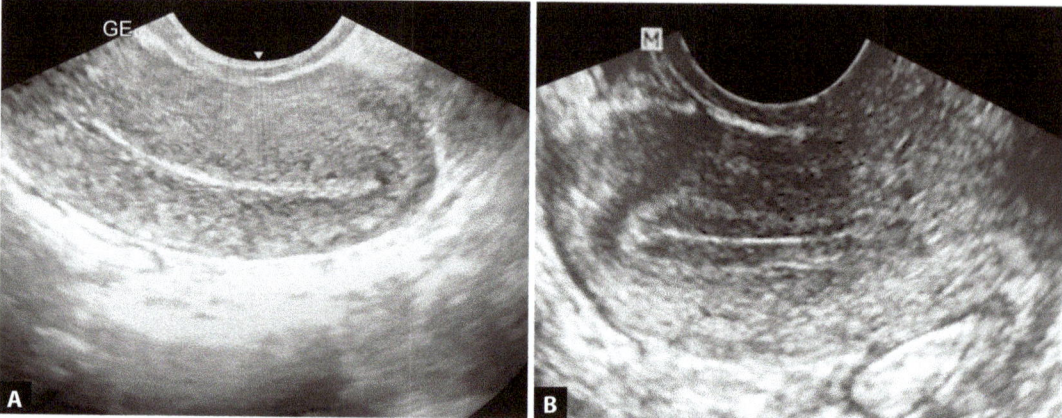

Figs. 7A and B: (A) Thin endometrium post-menses; (B) Grade C multilayered triple—line endometrium.

Grade C: Multilayered 'triple-line' endometrium consisting of prominent outer and central hyperechogenic line and inner hypoechogenic region **(Fig. 7B)**.

Common pathologies of endometrium are endometrial hyperplasia, polyps, synechiae, adhesion, endometritis.

Endometritis

Acute: It presents as thick isoechoic endometrium with disruption of functional zone. Fluid can be seen in the cavity. Chronic endometritis present as persistently thin avascular endometrium with disrupted functional zone, calcification in adnexa can be present.

Endometrial Polyps (Fig. 8)

- Solid echogenic lesion within the cavity.
- Best time to visualize is the pre-ovulatory phase.
- Polyps have single feeding vessel mostly.
- Polyp can be differentiated from submucosal fibroid because fibroid is mostly hypoechoic, well-demonstrated while polyp is hyperechoic.

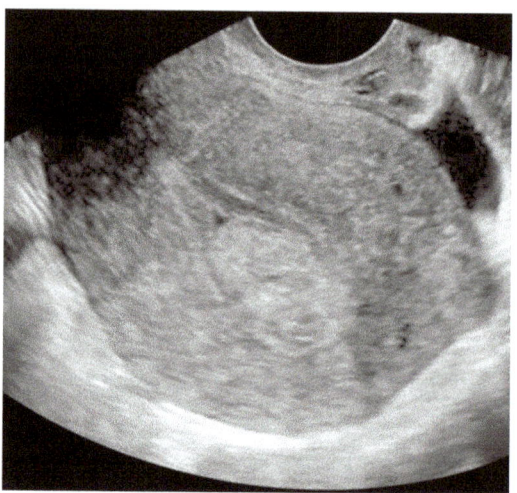

Fig. 8: Endometrial polyp.

Synechiae/Adhesions

Thin endometrium or absence of uniform endometrial lining is suggestive of intrauterine adhesion. It can be seen as lines bridging between layers of endometrium **(Fig. 9)**.

Adnexa

It includes:
- Ovarian/tubovarian lesion
- Pavaovarian, peritoneal cyst.

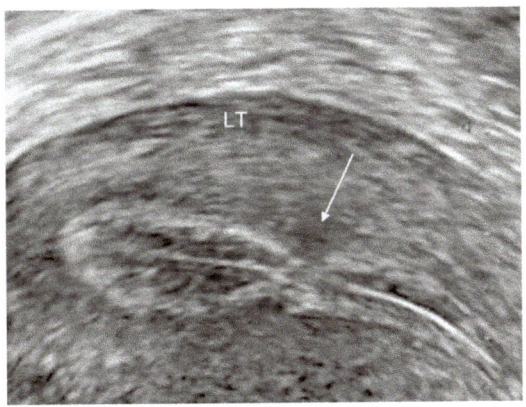

Fig. 9: Synechiae.

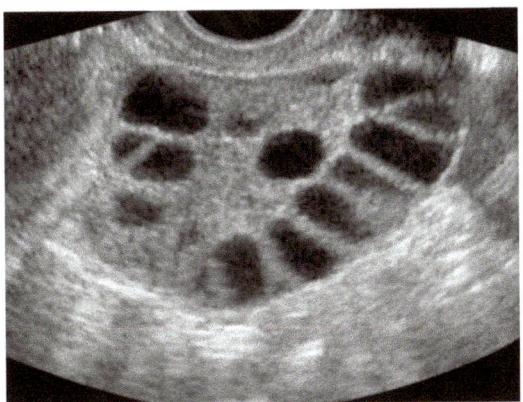

Fig. 10: Polycystic ovarian disease.

EVALUATION OF OVARIES

Evaluation of ovaries is an integral part of baseline scan. Baseline scan include the assessment of ovarian reserves. According to which there can be polycystic ovary, normal ovary, low ovarian reserve. Ovarian assessment consists of measurement of ovarian diameter, ovarian volume and AFC.

Antral Follicular Count

- It is the number of follicles 2–10 mm on D2/D3 of cycle.
- It is the test for assessment of poor ovarian reserve.
- It has good correlation with AMH and is useful for deciding the stimulation protocol for patients.
- It can help in predicting Ovarian hyperstimulation syndrome (OHSS) also.

POLYCYSTIC OVARIAN DISEASE (PCOD)

Rotterdam's criteria for polycystic ovaries include >12 follicular of 2–9 mm is one or both ovaries, increased volume >10 mL is suggestive PCOD. Apart from this increase stroma is a specific indicator of hyperandrogenism. The ratio of stromal area/ovarian area can determine ovarian hyperandrogenism **(Fig. 10)**.

LESIONS OF OVARIES

- Clear cysts
- Cyst with septum or internal echogenicity
- Solid lesions
- Complex cyst solid with cystic lesions

Clear Cyst

Follicular cyst: If the growing follicles does not rupture and it grows beyond 25 mm and persists in the luteal phase of cycle or even is subsequent cycle. It has scanty and high resistance flow. Sometimes there is a large cyst of >5 cm with no flow in Doppler. They are simple cyst and may need aspiration.

Cyst with Internal Echogenicity

All these have thick shaggy wall with internal echogenicity.
- Corpus luteum
- Hemorrhagic cyst
- Luteinized unruptured cyst
- Endometrioma

Corpus Luteum

It has thick, crenulated walls. It has heterogeneous echogenic content with or without septae. Doppler shows ring of color with low resistance RI <0.5

Endometrioma (Fig. 11)

Features are:
- Unilocular cyst with ground-glass appearance
- Thick shaggy wall without septa
- Linear echogenic flex in the wall
- Pain on pressure with the probe
- On Doppler, scattered vascularity with moderate vascular impedance.[7]

Solid Lesions

Fibroma is the most common lesion in this group. It is well-defined round oval lesion with echogenicity like that of a fibroid, hypoechoic, homogeneous but may be heterogeneous and may have calcification. Fibroma and fibroids can be differentiated by tracing the blood supply. Fibromas are often bilateral and may be associated with ascites and pleural effusion, the complication is known as Meigs's syndrome.

Ovarian torsion also has solid looking ovary in which the stroma is hypoechoic and peripherally placed, vascularity may or may not be present. Twisting of vessels gives the definitive sign known as Whirlpool sign.[8]

Complex Lesions with Solid Cystic Areas

Dermoid (Fig. 12)

- Dermoid cyst presents as solid hyperechoic, heterogeneous mass with mixed pattern area as they may contain calcification, hair, fat and teeth.
- Well-defined lesions with thick wall, low level echoes, fluid-filled levels,

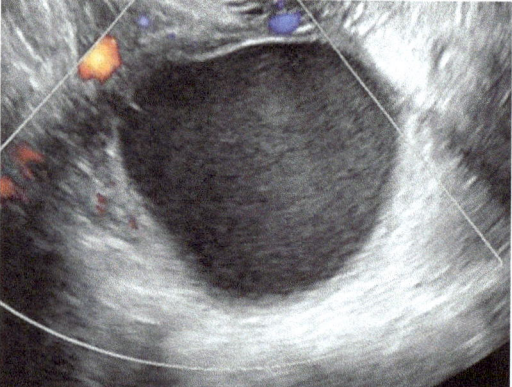

Fig. 11: Endometrial cyst containing homogeneous echoes and no internal vascularity.

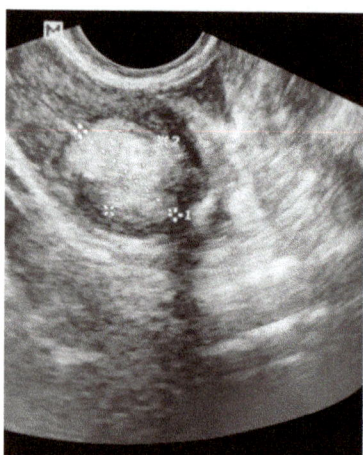
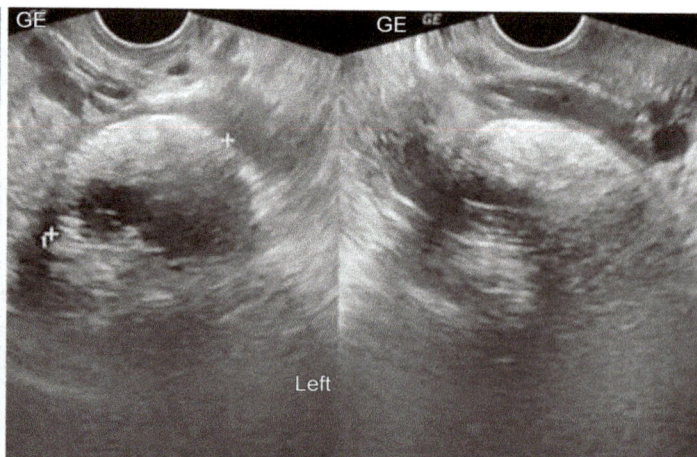

Fig. 12: Bilateral dermoid cysts.

hyperechoic lines due to hair, calcified echoes because of presence of teeth with posterior shadowing.
- There are regional bright echoes due to fat or hair clumps.
- Mostly they are avascular.

TUBAL LESIONS

- The most common tubal lesions are inflammatory in origin. Inflammation of fallopian tubes is known as salpingitis.
- This causes thickened fallopian tube, hydrosalpinx which appear as tubular cystic structure separate from the ovary. As the fallopian tube dilates it often develops as S, U, V, C or serpiginous shape **(Fig. 13B and Fig. 15)**.
- *Waist sign* consists of opposed indentation in the wall, usually observed at the junction of the ampullary portion of the tube **(Fig. 14)**.
- *Cogwheel sign:* Incomplete septation and internal projections due to thickened endosalpingeal fold along with thickened wall of tube usually seen in acute inflammation **(Fig. 13A)**.
- *Beads on string sign:* In chronic inflammation when tube walls become thinner and multiple mural-based echogenic nodules due to endosalpingeal fold thickening resulting in appearance of *Beads-on-a-String* **(Fig. 14)**.

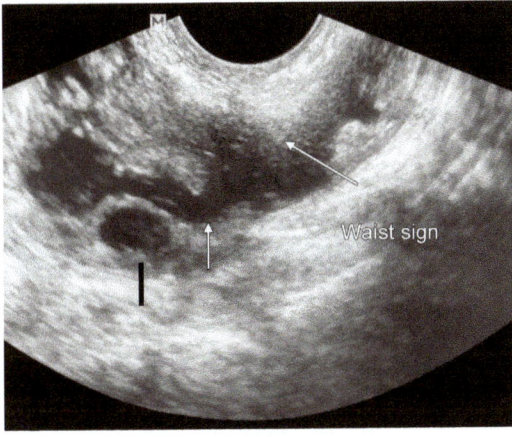

Fig. 14: Beads in a string, waist sign and incomplete septation.

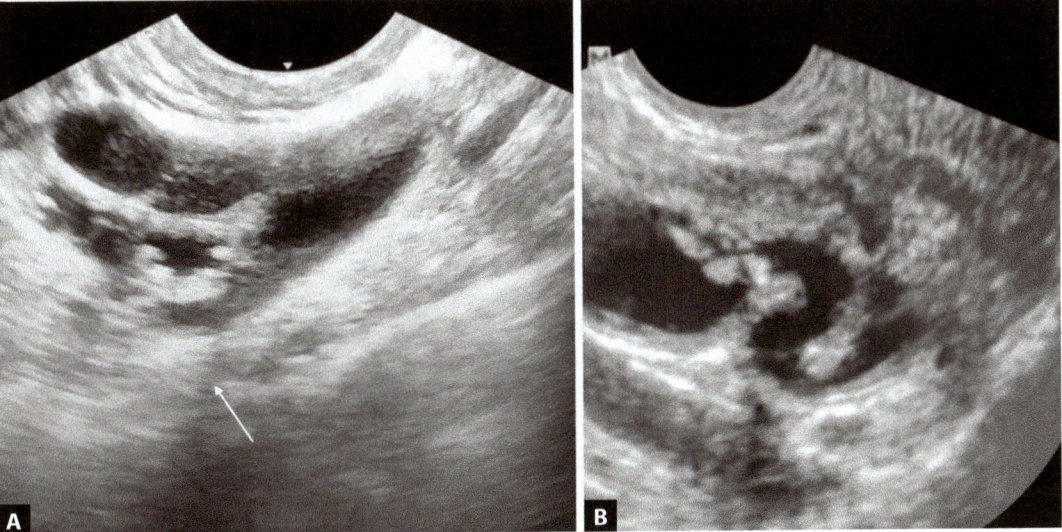

Figs. 13A and B: (A) Cogwheel sign; (B) Serpiginous or S-shaped hydrosalpinx.

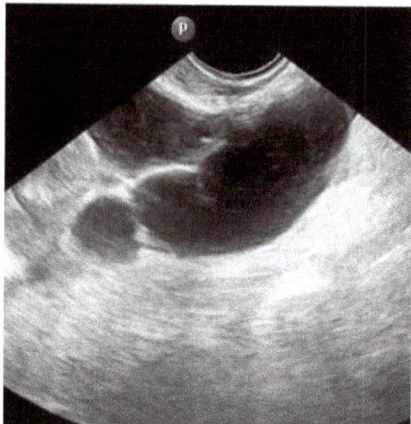

Fig. 15: Hydrosalpinx - Tubular, Cystic Fluid filled Structure in adnexa

Sonographic markers for the tubal inflammation[9]		
	Acute	Chronic
Thickened wall of tube (≥5 mm)	++	–
Cogwheel sign	++	–
Beads-on-a-String appearance (Flattened/fibrotic endosalpingeal folds 2–3 mm hyperechoic nodules on cross-section of fluid-filled structure)	–	+
Tubo-ovarian complex	+	–
Fluid in cul-de-sec	+	+/–

■ MONITORING OF CYCLE

Assessment of Follicle

- Ultrasonography is used to assess the direct effects of stimulatory drugs on the ovaries in ovarian stimulation protocols. It is necessary to individualize the stimulation protocol to get the desired number of oocytes and balance it against the risk of OHSS.
- Ovarian stimulation is monitored by manual counting of the follicles. Follicular diameter is measured by taking the mean of two perpendicular diameters. The rate of growth of individual follicles is useful in predicting ovulation and the risk of ovarian hyperstimulation than follicle diameter alone.
- The usual growth rate is 1.5 mm/day irrespective of whether they develop during a natural or a stimulated cycle.
- *Characteristics of a mature follicle:*
  - Size: 16–18 mm
  - Thin walls
  - Round in shape
  - No echogenicities in the lumen
  - Cumulus-like shadow (develops 36 hours before rupture)
- *Doppler features of a mature follicle:*

Blood flow in a follicle	
Blood flow covered (in a single cross area slice) (%)	Grade of vascularity
<25	1
25–30	2
50–75	3
>75	4

- *Resistivity index (RI):* 0.4–0.48
- Peak systolic velocity (PSV) greater than 10 cm/s in at least one grade 3–4 follicle predicted a pregnancy with sensitivity of 91%.[10]
- Decreased blood flow to the follicle signifies increased oocyte hypoxia and increased chances of chromosomal abnormalities.
- Human chorionic gonadotropin is usually administered when there is minimum one follicle of 16–18 mm in size.

Signs of ovulation:
- Irregular or disappearance of pre-existing follicle
- Presence of corpus luteum with vascular ring
- Free fluid in pouch of Douglas (POD)
- Corresponding hyperechogenic endometrium.

ENDOMETRIAL THICKNESS

In stimulated cycles, endometrium increases 1.9 mm between day 7 and 9 of stimulation, 0.9 between day 9 and 11, 0.6 mm between day 12 and day of hCG administration. Endometrial thickness of >7 mm is associated with higher pregnancy rate.[11]

ENDOMETRIAL VASCULARITY

A good blood supply towards the endometrium is usually considered to be an essential requirement for implantation and therefore assessment of endometrial blood flow in IVF treatment is very important.

Uterine blood flow, as measured by color Doppler is measured at the uterine artery and their ascending branches, is a suggested physiological parameter to assess receptivity.

Steer et al. demonstrates that the patients with a low uterine artery PI on the day of embryo transfer were more likely to conceive than those with a high PI. In this series, no one with PI >3.0 conceived.[12]

On Doppler, the vascularity is classified by Applebaum.[13] Measurement is done in the sagittal plane.

Zone 1: Blood vessels reaching endometrial-myometrial junction surrounding the endometrium. A 2 mm thick area surrounding the hyperechoic outer layer of endometrium.

Zone 2: Blood vessels reaching hyperechoic endometrial edge (hyperechoic outer layer of endometrium).

Zone 3: Blood vessel reaching internal endometrial hypoechoic zone.

Zone 4: Blood vessel reaching endometrial cavity homogeneous hyperechogenic in luteal phase **(Fig. 16)**.

Vascularity in Zone 3 and 4 are associated with successful embryo implantation.

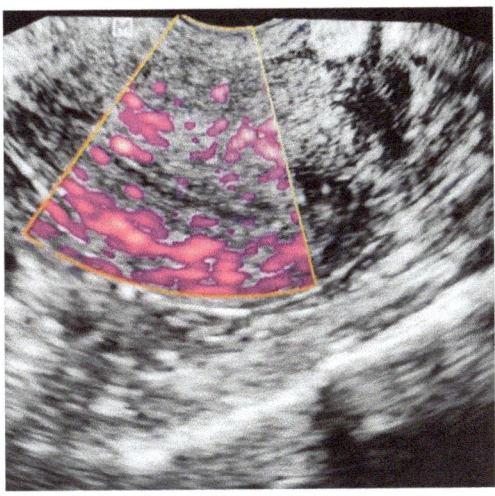

Fig. 16: Vascularity in zone 4.

UTERINE BIOPHYSICAL SCORE AND THE UTERINE SCORING SYSTEM FOR REPRODUCTION (USSR)

Uterine biophysical profile (UBP) is the 7 point scale noted in mid cycle to confirm preparedness of endometrium and predictors of implantation. The Uterine scoring system includes evaluation of following parameters:[14]

- Endometrial thickness in greatest AP dimension of 7 mm or greater
- A layered ("5 line") appearance to the endometrium
- Blood flow within zone 3 using color Doppler technique
- Myometrial contraction causing a wave-like motion of the endometrium (3 contractions in 2 min)
- Uterine arterial blood flow, as measured by PI, less than 3.0
- Homogeneous myometrial echogenicity
- Myometrial blood flow seen on gray scale examination (internal to the arcuate vessels).

ULTRASONOGRAPHY-GUIDED OOCYTE RETRIEVAL IN ART

In ART, oocyte retrieval is done under TVS guidance. An 18G needle is introduced through a guide attached to TVS probe. Echogenic needle tip is visible when introduced. Follicular fluid is aspirated with pressure of 110–120 mm Hg. Complications such as pelvic infection, injury to iliac vessel are rarely seen.

EMBRYO TRANSFER

After visualizing the cervix, mucus is removed. Transabdominal probe is placed suprapubically on the lower abdomen. Partially filled bladder facilitate better imaging. The outer embryo transfer catheter tip is visualized and positioned at the internal os. The inner catheter loaded with media droplet containing the embryos and small air columns to make the tip visible and to avoid accidental embryo spillage, is inserted through the outer catheter into the endometrial cavity. It is slowly and gently pushed from the transfer catheter into the uterine cavity. There is currently no consensus regarding the optimal position of embryo transfer within the uterine cavity but 1–2 cm below the fundus is considered best by most clinicians.[15]

CONCLUSION

Ultrasonography (USG) is the most acceptable, noninvasive, reliable mode of investigation. Ultrasonography has become an indispensable tool not only for gynecological infertility work-up but also for monitoring and treating infertility patients. TVS sonography should be the primary investigation modality for infertile patients.

Color Doppler and 3D ultrasonography are recent developments which have proven their usefulness and have given promising possibilities for the future.

REFERENCES

1. Bazot M, Darai E. Role of transvaginal sonography and magnetic resonance imaging in the diagnosing of uterine adenomyosis. Fertil Steril. 2018;109(3):389-97.
2. Bermejo C, Martinez P Ten, Cantarero D Diaz, et al. Three- dimensional ultrasound in the diagnosis of Müllerian duct anomalies and concordance with magnetic resonance imaging. Ultrasound in Obstetrics and Gynaecology.2010;35(5):593-601.
3. Raga F, Bonilla-Musoles F, Blanes J, Osborne NG. Congenital Müllerian anomalies: diagnostic accuracy of three-dimensional ultrasound. Fertil Steril. 1996;65(3):523-8.
4. Ayida G, Harris P, Kennedy S, et al. Hysterosalpingo-contrast sonography (HyCoSy) using Echovist-200 in the outpatient investigation of infertility patients. Br J Radiol. 1996;69:910-3.
5. Alcazar JL. Transvaginal color Doppler in patients with ovarian endometriomas and pelvic pain. Hum Gynecol.2001;16 (16):2672-5.
6. Gonen Y, et al. Prediction of implantation by the sonographic appearance of the endometrium during controlled ovarian stimulation for in vitro fertilization (IVF). J In Vitro Fert Embryo Transf. 1990;7(3):146-52.
7. Panchal S, Nagori C. Doppler in Myometrial Lesions. Donald School Journal of Ultrasound in Obstetrics and Gynecology, 2019
8. Sibal M. Follicular ring sign: a simple sonographic sign for early diagnosis of ovarian torsion. J Ultrasound Med. 2012; 31(11):1803-9.
9. Panchal S, et al. Transvaginal Ultrasound and Doppler in Infertility: Principles and Practice of Assisted Reproductive Technology, Vol 1. 405-434.

10. Vetman-Verhulsy SM, Chlen BJ, Hughes E, et al. Intrauterine insemination for unexplained subfertility. Cochrane Database Syst Rev. 2012;Issue (Art. No:CD001838).
11. Bassil S. Changes in endometrial thickness, width, length and pattern in predicting pregnancy outcome during ovarian stimulation in in vitro fertilization. Ultrasound Obstet Gynecol. 2001;18:258-63.
12. Steer CV, Campbell S, et al. The use of transvaginal color flow imaging after in vitro fertilization to identify optimum uterine conditions before embryo transfer. Fertil Steril. 1992;57(2):372-6.
13. Appelbaum Michael. The Uterine Biophysical Profile (UBP). Endosonography in Obstetrics and Gynecology (Ed). Gautam Allahabadia, Rotunda Medical Technologies (P) Ltd, Mumbai, India.1997;343 -52.
14. FOGSI Update in Obstetrics & Gynecology, Vol 2, 2022.
15. IFFS 2016 Pre-congress Proceedings

Management of Tubal Factor in Fertility

CHAPTER 7

Anu Agarwal, Shikha Sachan

■ INTRODUCTION

Tubal factor infertility accounts for about 25 to 30% of all cases.

The fallopian tube plays an important role in the mechanical transport and physiological sustenance of gametes and early conceptus.

Causes

- Tubal obstruction or occlusion (proximal, distal unilateral or bilateral)[1]
- Endosalpingeal destruction[2]
- Periadenexal adhesion[3]
- Pelvic inflammatory disease (PID)[4]
- Endometriosis[5]
- Ectopic pregnancy[6]
- Abdominal pelvic surgery, induced surgical abortions, septic abortion.[7]

Pelvic Inflammatory Disease (PID)

- PID is responsible for more than 50% of the cases and usually affects tubes at multiple sites.[8] In most cases, infection is ascending, and *Chlamydia trachomatis* and *Neisseria gonorrhea* or common organisms with increased incidence.
- Nearly 10% of all cervical infections ascend to the upper genital tract leading to salpingitis.
- In countries like India where *Mycobacterium tuberculosis* is endemic, genital tuberculosis is one of the common causes of tubal inflammatory disease.
- Fallopian tubes are involved in almost all patients with genital tuberculosis causing congestion, flimsy adhesions, plastic adhesions, hydrosalpinx, pyosalpinx and tuboovarian masses.

■ EVALUATION OF TUBAL INFERTILITY

- Hysterosalpingography (HSG)
- TVS and hysterosalpingo-contrast sonography (HyCoSy)
- Chlamydia antibody testing (CAT)
- Laproscopy
- Hysteroscopy
- Falloposcopy
- Salpingoscopy
- Fertiloscopy
- Salpingography
- Computed tomography (CT) and virtual HSG
- MRI.

Hysterosalpingography

Radiographic evaluation of the uterus and fallopian tubes. Two contraindications are:
1. Pregnancy
2. Active pelvic infection

Time

6 to 10 days of the menstrual cycle (women were advised to take non-steroidal anti-inflammatory drugs, 1 hour prior to the procedure)

Complications of HSG

- Bleeding, infection, cramping pain
- Reaction to the contrast material (uncommon due to the use of low osmolar non-ionic contrast agent)
- Perforation of the uterus or fallopian tube (extremely infrequent complication). The fallopian tube should appear as thin lines that widen in the ampullary portion tubal abnormalities seen in an HSG can be:
  - Congenital
  - *Spasm:* One or both tubes may not fill beyond the interstitial portion.
  - Occlusion or infection
  - *Salpingitis isthmic nodosa (SIN):* Associated with infertility, PID and occasionally ectopic pregnancy. SIN is a small outpouching or diverticulum from the isthmic portion of the fallopian tube.
  - Peritubal adhesions—prevents contrast, material from flowing freely around the bowel loops and most commonly manifest as loculation of contrast material around the ampullary portion of the tube.
  - *Tubal polyps:* Smooth, rounded, filling defect without concomitant dilatation or tubal occlusion.

Tubal Tuberculosis

- X-ray shows calcification of the fallopian tube or ovaries.
- Caseous ulceration of the mucosa of the tube produces an irregular contour of mucosa leading to an irregular contour of the lumen of the tube.
- *Tufted appearance*: Diverticular cavities surround the ampulla and give this appearance.
- *Isthmic diverticula resembling SIN*: Multiple constrictions along the course of the fallopian tube can form because of scarring and give rise to a *beaded appearance* and *rigid pipe appearance*.

Accuracy:

- The negative predictive value of HSG for detecting patency or occlusion for the right and left fallopian tubes was 92.08% and 95.44% respectively. The positive predictive value of HSG for detecting patency or occlusion for both tubes was 87.2%.
- HSG may have a therapeutic effect because of tubal flushing.

Ultrasound Evaluation of the Fallopian Tube

The normal fallopian tube can occasionally be visualized with TVS, especially when there is some fluid in the adnexal region and minimal pressure is exerted on the probe.

The normal fallopian tube appears solid, separate from the ovary and isoechoic to the uterus **(Fig. 1)**. The presence of para-tubal cyst also known as hydrated of Morgagni may

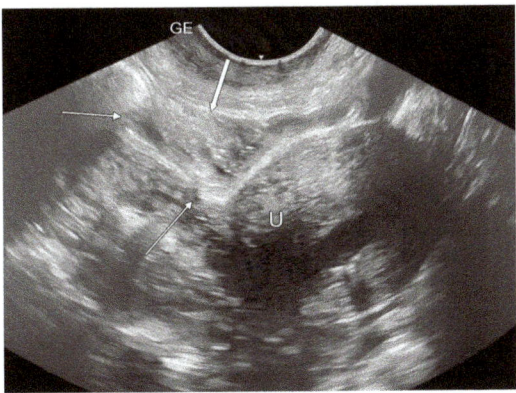

Fig. 1: Normal fallopian tube—arrows coursing from the cornua of the uterus (U). Note the more medial isthmic portion (thin arrows) of the tube is the thinnest segment, whereas the fimbriated end (thick arrows), which usually sits above the ovary, is the thickest segment.

Courtesy: Dr Anu Agarwal, Vansh Fertility and Test Tube Baby Centre, Varanasi, Uttar Pradesh, India.

help to localize the tubes (They are small, unilocular, simple cyst, located at the fimbrial end of the fallopian tube between the tube and ovary). An echogenic fat plane between cyst and ovary and the absence of a surrounding rim of ovarian parenchyma differentiate a para tubal cyst from exophytic ovarian tissue. So to conclude, both normal and abnormal tubes can be identified using ultrasound. Hydrosalpinx, pyosalpinx, or hematosalpinx demonstrate a variety of classic sonographic signs that can be used to differentiate a cystic mass of tubal origin from ovarian and other pelvic causes.

These signs are:
- Waist sign
- Incomplete septation sign
- Cogwheel sign
- Beads on a string sign
- Serpiginous or S-shaped hydrosalpinx.

Saline infusion sonography (SIS): Injection of saline agitated with air bubbles can confirm tubal patency. The bubbles are fairly evanescent.

Accumulation of free fluid in the peritoneal cavity during the routine SIS implies the patency of at least one fallopian tube.

Hysterosalpingography Contrast

Sonography contrast agent Echovist-200 can be used to obtain a real-time image of hyperechoic flow through the fallopian tube.

Laparoscopy

Laparoscopy with chromopertubation is the Gold standard method for evaluating tubal patency.

Hysteroscopy

Hysteroscopic tubal catheterization is an effective therapeutic method in patience with proximal tubal occlusion.

Falloposcopy

Used to characterize normal and abnormal epithelial change, document endotubal lesions, identification of the segmental location of tubal pathology.

Salpingoscopy

Visual inspection of the ampullary mucosa during either laparotomy or laparoscopy.

MRI

Aids in non-invasive assessment of tubal dilatation and peritubal disease.

Dilated fallopian tube manifests as fluid-filled ducts appearing as retort, sausage, C or S- shaped cystic masses at MRI.

General Considerations

Of all the reproductive organs, fallopian tube plays an important role in fertilization and have a very delicate structure. It is to be noted that tubal blockage is many a times secondary consequence of a primary pathology like PID, chlamydia infection, etc. Management of tubal blockage has to be individualized where if appropriately chosen surgery in expert hands can benefit a number of patients, while if selection is not made judiciously it can increase the risk of ectopic pregnancy. IVF is a boon for people with tubal diseases such as hydrosalpinx, where surgical procedures such as tubal clipping have added advantage.

Counseling patients with tubal infertility regarding corrective surgery vs. IVF plays a very important role in management as we help the patient to make a guided choice according to various factors.

The various factors to be considered are:
- *Age of the patient:* Surgery usually benefits younger age group and those with preserved tubal anatomy, but in cases of

tubal ligation surgery even in later years in expert hands proves to be beneficial.
- Ovarian reserve
- Prior fertility
- Number of children desired
- Site and extent of tubal disease
- Presence of other infertility factors
- Experience of the surgeon
- Success rates of IVF program
- Patient preference
- Religious belief
- Cost
- Insurance reimbursement.

The various advantages and disadvantages of tubal surgery and IVF should be discussed with the patient to help her choose her choice of procedure. The main advantages and disadvantages are:

Advantages of IVF in Tubal Pathologies

Good per cycle success rates as the treatment are tailored according to other parameters of the patient and it is less invasive than surgical procedures,[9] also the anesthetic and surgical complications associated with surgical procedures are not seen here.

Disadvantages of IVF in Tubal Pathologies

- Cost (especially if >1 cycle is required)
- Need for frequent injections
- Monitoring for several weeks
- Risk of multiple pregnancies
- Risk of ovarian hyperstimulation syndrome.

Advantages of Tubal Surgery

- One-time, minimally invasive OPD procedure
- The patient is free to try conception every month without any other further intervention or medication
- May conceive more than once.

Disadvantages of Tubal Surgery

- Risk of surgical complications
- Postoperative discomfort
- The risk of ectopic pregnancy increased.

To have better pregnancy rates and to reduce the risks like tube damage and ectopic, surgeries should be performed by experienced laparoscopic surgeon expert in microsurgical techniques.

The ideal patient for tubal surgery is:
- Young
- Has no other significant infertility factors
- Has tubal anatomy, i.e., amenable to repair.

Tuboplasty

Tuboplasty or tubal microsurgery is chosen procedure for young women with tubal blockage and prior tubal sterilization. Several tuboplasty procedures have been performed with successful pregnancy rates of 50–60% for the isthmic blockage to 27% for fimbrial surgery. Salpingectomy or clipping of large hydrosalpinx is also recommended procedure before planning the patient for IVF.[9] The various tuboplasty procedures are:[10]
- Tubocornual anastomosis
- Tubotubal anastomosis
- Salpingostomy
- Adhesiolysis (Salpingo-ovariolysis)
- Fimbrioplasty
- Cornual implantation.

Tubal Ligation Reversal

- Microsurgical anastomosis is the preferred method for tubal ligation reversal.
- Tubal ligation is reversed by trying to open the occluded ends of the cut/occluded proximal and distal ends and uniting them with fine sutures. This is performed using microsurgical techniques and under magnification.

- Anastomoses is typically achieved with a 2-layer technique including 4 interrupted sutures placed in the muscular followed by the re-approximation of the overlying serosa.
- The reversal of sterilization procedures performed with rings or clips results in higher pregnancy rates than for sterilization performed via ligation/resection or coagulation.
- Despite comparable pregnancy and ectopic rates, case times for minimally invasive tubal reversal are longer than an open approach.
- The main challenge in laparoscopic anastomoses is the technical demands of laparoscopic suturing.
- Surgeons facile with laparoscopic suturing and who have experience and training in tubal microsurgery should attempt this procedure.
- Other prognostic factors which are thought to predict success include:
  - Final tube length
  - Site of tubal re-approximation, i.e., isthmic-isthmic reversals may have greater success than ampullary or cornual segments.
- Surgeons may wish to defer the reversal procedures in instances of:
  - Final tubal length <4 cm
  - Significant tubo-ovarian adhesions
  - Advanced endometriosis
  - Recognized significant male factor infertility.

Surgical treatment is again divided according to the site of tubal blockage:
- Proximal tubal blockage
- Distal tubal blockage.

Under fluoroscopic guidance using a coaxial catheter system or with the help of hysteroscopy, it is always better to have a laparoscopic confirmation to rule out inadvertent cannulation.

An outer catheter is passed through the uterotubal ostium, and the site of blockage is again confirmed by a selective salpingogram.[11] If the tubal blockage is confirmed, a flexible guidewire through a small inner catheter is advanced through the proximal tube. By this cannulation, even after gentle pressure, if the obstruction is not overcome, then the procedure is terminated and a true anatomic occlusion is performed.[11] This procedure is most successful in proximal tubal obstruction in young women with no other significant infertility factors. On the other hand, IVF would be the preferred treatment for proximal tubal blockage in older women and in the presence of significant male factor infertility.

Distal Tubal Disease

Distal tubal diseases include hydrosalpinges, fimbrial phimosis, and peritubular adhesions. Surgery has to be cautiously chosen in this category. There are several pointers for this like:

Patients with good prognosis after surgery have:
- Limited flimsy adnexal adhesions
- Mildly dilated tubes <3 cm
- With thin and pliable walls
- Lush endosalpinx with preservation of mucosal folds.

Patients having poor prognosis have:
- Extensive dense peritubal adhesions
- Largely dilated tubes with thick fibrotic walls
- Sparse or absent luminal mucosa.

Laparoscopic fimbrioplasty or neosalpingostomy is recommended for the treatment of mild hydrosalpinges in young women with no other significant infertility factors. Laparoscopic salpingectomy should be used for proximal tubal occlusion in cases of surgically irreparable hydrosalpinges to improve IVF pregnancy rates. Aspiration of hydrosalpinx with or without sclerotherapy may be superior to no treatment at all, but further studies are needed.

REFERENCES

1. Farhi J, Ben-Haroush A. Distribution of causes of infertility in patients attending primary fertility clinics in Israel. IAMJ. 2011;13:51-4.
2. Omurtag K, Grindler NM, Roehi K.A. Wright Bates G, Beltsos AN, Odenm RR, Jungheim ES. How do members of the Society for Reproductive Endocrinology and Infertility and the Society of Reproductive Surgeons evaluate, define and manage hydrosalpinges. Fertil Steril. 2012;97(5) doi:10.1016/j.fertnstert.2012.02.026. [PMC free article].
3. Zou SE, Jin Y, Ko YL, Zhu J. A new classification system for pregnancy prognosis of tubal factor infertility. Int J Clin Exp Med. 2014;7(5):1410-16. [PMC free article].
4. Malhotra M. Sood S, Mukherjee A, Muralidhar S, Bala M. Genital *Chlamydia trachomatis:* an update. Indian J Med Res. 2013;138(3):303-16. [PMC free article].
5. Singh N, Lata K, Naha M, Malhotra N, Tiwari A, Vanamail P. Effect of endometriosis on implantation rates when compared to tubal factor in fresh non donor in vitro fertilization cycle. J Hum Reprod Sci. 2014;7(2):143-7. [PMC free article].
6. Junior JE, Han KK, Camano L. Tubal patency following surgical and clinical treatment of ectopic pregnancy. Sao Paolo Med J. 2006;124(5):264-6.
7. Minh PN, Vihn NQ, Tuong HM, Danh MTC, Lan VTN, Trong DMH, Hai HT, Quoc NT, Hanh TLM, Dong LK, Goto A. A case-control study on the relationship between induced abortion and secondary tubal infertility in Vietnam. Fukushima J Med Sci. 2002;48(1):15-25.
8. Honore GM, Holden AE, Schenken RS. Pathophysiology and management of proximal tubal blockage. Fertil Steril. 1999;71(5):785-95.
9. Dun EC, Nezhat CH. (2012). Tubal factor infertility diagnosis and management in the era of assisted reproductive technology. Obstetrics and Gynecology Clinics of North America. 2012;39:551-66. 10.1016/j.ogc.2012.09.006.
10. Ambildhuke K, Pajai S, Chimegave A, et al. (November 01, 2022). A review of tubal factors affecting fertility and its management. Cureus. 14(11):e30990. doi:10.7759/ cureus.30990
11. The Practice Committee of the American Society for Reproductive Medicine. Role of tubal surgery in the era of assisted reproductive technology: a committee opinion. Fertility and Sterility® Vol. 115, No. 5, May 2021 0015-0282/$36.00 Copyright© 2021 American Society for Reproductive Medicine, Published by Elsevier Inc. https://doi.org/10.1016/j.fertnstert.2021.01.051.

CHAPTER 8

Anovulatory Infertility

Rehana Najam, Jaideep Malhotra

■ INTRODUCTION

Infertility has become one of the leading causes for consultation in gynecological OPD. Among the various factors responsible for female subfertility, ovarian factors especially chronic anovulation form one large spectrum in reproductive endocrinology. Anovulation accounts for infertility in 25% of subfertile women.[1,2] Anovulation can be one of the earliest symptoms of functional or organic hypothalamic diseases, pituitary disease, or inappropriate feedback by the peripheral hormones and primary ovarian insufficiency.[2]

■ DEFINITION

Anovulation per se is characterized by failure to release a mature oocyte on a regular monthly basis. Anovulation presents various clinical manifestations that include amenorrhea, infertility, hirsutism, and menstrual irregularities.[3]

CLASSIFICATION AND ETIOLOGICAL PERSPECTIVES

Infertility caused by anovulation can be classified according to deficiency of the hypothalamic-pituitary-ovarian axis (HPO axis) at different levels.[4]

Causes of anovulation according to WHO classification

Hypogonadotropic hypogonadism (WHO Group I)
- Functional hypothalamic dysfunction (e.g., excessive exercise, overstress, weight loss such as in anorexia nervosa, drug intake, iatrogenic)
- Pan-pituitary infarct as in Sheehan's syndrome, pituitary tumor
- Kallmann syndrome
- Idiopathic hypogonadotropic hypogonadism

Normogonadotropic normogonadism (WHO Group II)
Polycystic ovary syndrome (PCOS)

Hypergonadotropic hypogonadism (WHO Group III)
- Iatrogenic as in post-radiotherapy, surgical menopause or chemotherapy
- Genetic disorder like Turner syndrome
- Infectious causes such as mumps and oophoritis
- Autoimmune causes
- Idiopathic
- Other various endocrinopathies such as thyroid disorder, including hyperpro lactinemia, congenital adrenal hyperplasia, ovarian and adrenal tumor.

Hypogonadotropic Hypogonadism Causes (WHO Group I)

The main feature of hypogonadotropic hypogonadism is that there is no luteinizing hormone (LH) and FSH release as there is no production of these hormones by pituitary.

There is physiological decrease in production of gonadotropin-releasing hormone (GnRH) from hypothalamus which causes amenorrhea. The most common cause is over-exercising usually seen in athletes and other common cause is being underweight with low body mass index (BMI).

Normogonadotropic Normogonadism (WHO Group II)

Polycystic Ovary Syndrome

Accounts for 70% of infertility occurring due to anovulation. In PCOS, the excess production of androgens within the ovary results in the recruitment of increased numbers of preovulatory follicles. No dominant follicle is produced. In insulin, resistance is the main pathophysiological abnormality and is seen in only 10–15% of PCOS women who are slim and 20–40% of PCOS women are obese.[5] According to Rotterdam 2003 criteria, PCOS is defined as the presence of oligo- or anovulation, clinical and/or biochemical signs of hyperandrogenism or polycystic ovaries (PCO) after excluding related disorders such as thyroid disorders, hyperprolactinemia, congenital adrenal hyperplasia.[6]

If any two of the above features are present, she is diagnosed to have PCOS.

Obesity and Anovulation

In obese women, peripheral conversion of androgens to estrogens increase, causing imbalance in the secretion of gonadotropins. There is also decrease the sex hormone-binding globulin in the blood, along with decrease in the growth hormone secretion and also decrease in insulin-like growth factor binding proteins and increase in leptin levels, causing alteration in the HPO axis.

Hypergonadotropic Hypogonadism (Ovarian Failure) (WHO III Group)

Premature Ovarian Failure

This condition cannot be reversed. This can only be treated by in vitro fertilization (IVF) with donor oocytes. Hormone replacement therapy is given for menopause symptoms and to prevent loss of bone density.

Genetic Abnormalities

- Turner syndrome (45, X) in which the ovaries are underdeveloped (Streak) and so there is primary ovarian failure.
- Androgen insensitivity syndrome also called testicular feminization can cause primary amenorrhea.

■ DIAGNOSIS

History and Physical Examination

Women with ovulatory disorder present with a history of infertility. Detailed Clinical history enquiring about menstrual cycles duration, cyclicity, flow, prolonged cycles, amenorrhea, excessive cold or heat intolerance, primary or secondary weight gain, hirsutism, acne, discharge from the breast, headaches, treatment for pituitary tumors even history of drugs such as hormonal pills must be included.

A complete physical examination focusing on the secondary sexual characteristics, features of hyperandrogenism, galactorrhea and calculation of BMI, must be done.

Documentation of anovulation with specific biochemical and radiological tests such as serum progesterone on day 21 of less than 3 ng/mL, antral follicular count of less than 5–7 on day 2 of cycles but one may get more than 12–14 follicles in each ovary in cases of PCOS. One can also get follicular growth monitoring by USG.

Biochemical testing for thyroid, prolactin, and blood sugars in diabetic cases.

MANAGEMENT

Management must take into consideration a holistic approach including lifestyle change, psychological aspects and weight reduction correction of thyroid and prolactin levels.[6,7]

MEDICAL OPTIONS FOR OVULATION INDUCTION

1. Clomiphene Citrate (CC)

It is the treatment of choice for WHO group II anovulation. Through its antiestrogenic effect, it displaces endogenous estrogen from estrogen receptors in the hypothalamic-pituitary axis, this in turn reduces its negative feedback and hence increasing the secretion of endogenous GnRH and gonadotropins, which therefore induces ovulation.[7,8]

Before Starting Clomiphene Citrate

- Thyroid function tests should be normal.
- Serum prolactin should be normal.
- Male partners should be evaluated.
- Progesterone withdrawal bleeding should be present in otherwise amenorrhoic patient.
- Adrenal function should be normal.
- Tubal factors should be normal.

Contraindications

Large ovarian cyst >5 cm in diameter.
- Liver disease
- Hypogonadotropic hypogonadism
- Hypergonadotropic hypogonadism.

Treatment Regimens

The starting dose is 50 mg daily for 5 days and can go up to 150 mg/day. The treatment is usually started on day 2 after spontaneous or withdrawal bleeding otherwise. The ovulation rate is 73%, and pregnancy and live-birth rates are 36% and 29% per woman.[7]

Dose of clomiphene citrate and ovulation rate:
- American College of Obstetricians and Gynecologists (ACOG) recommendation depicts that CC can be used for a maximum of 12 months in a lifetime and for 6 months continuously. Therefore, monitoring for evidence of ovulation is a must when the patient is on CC.

Dose	Ovulation rate
50 mg	52%
100 mg	22%
150 mg	12%
200 mg	7%

- *Monitoring:*
  1. Serum progesterone in the mid-luteal phase if >3 ng/mL is evidence of ovulation. It is done to confirm ovulation with CC.
  2. If LH on days 8–9 is >10 IU/ML, the success rate is very low because of the poor quality of ova and embryo.
  3. Monitoring during CC treatment is a must because it can be used only for 3–6 months. The majority of conception occurs within the first 3 months.

Clomiphene Citrate + Antagonist

This makes a good combination in thin, lean PCOS patients where LH is tonical ly raised. It improves the quality of ovum and also the conception rates.

Ideal patients to start antagonist are those patients who are on clomiphene citrate therapy having LH level >10 IU/mL on day 8–9 of the cycle.

Antagonist is started when the size of follicles is 14 mm and is continued till the day of trigger.

Clomiphene Citrate + Metformin

In CC-resistant cases of PCOS when the metformin is combined with CC, it increases ovulation four to nine times than clomiphene alone.

It is logical to routinely use metformin with CC in obese women with PCOS and glucocorticoids as the first adjunct of choice for nonobese PCOS women failing to respond to CC.[9]

Clomiphene Citrate + Drilling

It is done in CC-resistant PCOS cases with the advantage of decreased multiple pregnancies and less OHSS.[10]

Clomiphene + Low-dose Aspirin

Aspirin may be used to increase the blood flow by vasodilatation which may counter the effects of stress in reducing pelvic blood flow.

2. Insulin-sensitizing Agents

Used to increase the insulin responsiveness in tissues, which reduces the hyperinsulinemic condition. This improves ovulatory function. Metformin, a biguanide, is the common insulin sensitizer used, the dose is 850 mg twice daily with meals.

3. Aromatase Inhibitors: Letrozole

Blocks the production of estrogen by hindering the conversion of androstenedione to estrone and testosterone to estradiol and the negative feedback to the hypothalamic-pituitary axis is decreased, causing increase in endogenous FSH secretion. It is used in ovulation induction in women with PCOS. Letrozole, a third-generation aromatase inhibitor is used for ovulation induction.

It is used in the dose of 2.5–5 mg per day for 5 days starting on the second day of spontaneous or induced bleeding or as a single dose of 20 mg on day 3 of the period.[11]

New Regimens

- *Extended letrozole therapy:* 2.5 mg letrozole is given from day 1 for 10 days in CC-resistant PCOS patients. It may produce more follicles and may give better pregnancy rates.
- *Letrozole step-up protocol:* 1, 2, 3, 4 tablets of 2.5 mg of letrozole are given respectively on day 2, 3, 4, and 5. This gives multifollicular development and a higher pregnancy rate.[12,13]

Letrozole + Gonadotropins

Letrozole + recombinant FSH (rFSH), a very useful combination for giving equivalent pregnancy rates like gonadotropins with the advantage that a lower number of ampoules are required.[14.]

Letrozole + Clomiphene Citrate

As both drugs have different mechanism of action, the combination of both may improve the ovulation rate than letrozole alone.[15]

Letrozole in a dose 2.5 mg and CC 50 mg from day 3 to 7 in PCOS patients. Patient who received both the drugs had a higher ovulation rate.

4. Gonadotropin-releasing Hormone

In hypogonadotropin, anovulation caused by hypothalamic dysfunction, GnRH is given for treatment but this is of no help in pituitary problem.

Gonadotropin

A combined preparation of both FSH and LH gives better outcome than only FSH in women with hypogonadotropic hypogonadism because LH activity is required for steroidogenesis in ovary to achieve optimal proliferation of endometrium.

Follicle Stimulating Hormone Preparations[16]

- *Human menopausal gonadotropins:* 75 IU of FSH and 75 IU of LH activity with human chorionic gonadotropins (hCG) which acts as LH surrogates.
- *Human menopausal gonadotropins (hMG) (highly purified):* 75 IU of FSH and 75 IU of LH with <5% of urinary proteins.
- Urinary FSH (uFSH) –75 IU of FSH and 1 IU of LH.
- FSH-HP-75 IU of FSH with <0.1 IU of LH and <1% of urinary proteins.
- *rFSH:* 75 IU of FSH and no LH activity.
- rFSH + recombinant LH (rLH) combination.

Different Regimens of Gonadotropin Therapy

1. Step-up protocol
2. Step-down protocol
3. Chronic low-dose protocol.

Step-up Protocol[15]

Started with 75 IU of FSH from day 5 for 5 days. An ultrasound scan is done on day 6 of stimulation. If this scan shows a follicle of 10–12 mm and there is a 2–3 mm increase in endometrial thickness, the same dose is continued till the follicle and endometrium become mature.

If there is no increase in size of follicle or not much change in endometrial thickness, the dose is doubled and the scan is repeated after 3 days. If the follicle and endometrium grows, the same dose is continued till the follicle and endometrium are mature; otherwise, the dose is further increased by 75 IU/day.

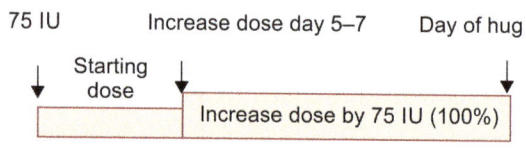

Step-down Protocol[17]

The step down protocol is very useful for poor responding ovaries or low reserve ovaries. According to this protocol, stimulation is started with a higher dose, i.e., 150–225 IU FSH from day 5 for 5 days. Once the follicle grows to 10–12 mm, the dose is reduced to 75–150 IU FSH; once the follicle size reaches to 14 mm, the dose is further reduced, if it was 150 IU or is continued with 75 IU FSH till follicle and endometrium matures.

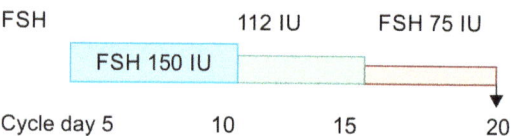

Chronic Low-dose Protocol[18,19]

The chronic low-dose protocol is very useful in PCOS patient. In this, stimulation is started with 75 IU of FSH and the same dose is continued for 14 days. If the follicle and endometrium grows, the same dose is continued till mature follicle and endometrium are achieved, otherwise the dose is increased by 37.5 IU for another 7 days.

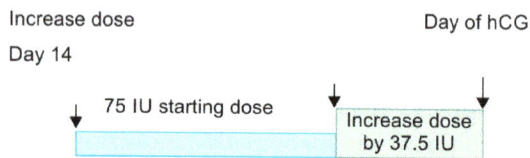

GONADOTROPIN-RELEASING HORMONE AGONIST[19,20]

Agonist are used for down regulation and this in IUI cycle only increases the requirement of gonadotropins, without increasing pregnancy rate.

GnRH agonist	Dose	Route
Decapeptyl	100–500 mg/day	SC
Triptorelin	3.75 mg depot	IM
Naperelin	400 mg BD	Nasal
Goserelin	3.6 mg/month	SC/implant
Buserelin	300–400 mg 200–500 mg	Intranasal SC
Leuprolide	0.5–1 mg daily 3.75 ng/month	SC/IM

GONADOTROPIN-RELEASING HORMONE AGONIST PROTOCOLS FOR ASSISTEDREPRODUCTIVE TECHNOLOGY

- Long protocol
- Short protocol
- Ultrashort protocol
- Microdose protocol.

Long Protocol[19]

Gonadotropin-releasing hormone agonist is started from mid-luteal phase, i.e., day 21 of the cycle. Leuprolide acetate 1 mg daily can be given to the patient oral depot preparation of 3.75 mg can be given. The 1 mg dose is continued till the patients get periods. The period comes when there is adequate downregulation. E2 level will be between 30 and 50 pg/mL at this time.

Gonadotropins are started from day 2 of menstruation. The dose is based on ultrasound parameters, anti-Müllerian hormone (AMH) levels or age and AMH together.

As the pituitary is already down regulated, the dose of GnRH is reduced to half in the daily dose protocol (0.25–0.5 mg daily). This dose is given till the day of ovulation trigger.

Pretreatment with oral contraceptive (OC) pills for 14 days prior to starting GnRHa can reduce the cyst formation without negative effect on pregnancy rates.

Downregulation can be confirmed by:
- Estradiol <30 pg/mL
- LH <2.5 IU/L
- Progesterone <2 ng/mL
- Endometrial thickness <4 mm.

Short Protocol[20]

In short protocol, 1 mg of leuprolide acetate is given daily from day 1 or 2 of the menstrual cycle. Gonadotropins are started from day 2 or day 3, i.e., 1 day after the agonist is started. Agonist is continued till the day of trigger with gonadotropins. This protocol is used for poor responders and the advantage is that the initial flare-up effect can be used for development of the follicles.

Ultrashort Protocol[22]

In this protocol, GnRH is started from day 1–2 of the menstruation in a dose of 0.5–1 mg/day. Given for 3 days only. Started from day 2 or 3, i.e., 1 day after GnRH is started.

Microdose Flare Protocol

Microdose flare protocol is the shortest protocol in which instead of 200 μg of daily dose only 50 μg is given daily.

Generic name	Trade name	Half life	Relative potency	Administration route	Recommended dose
Native GnRH			1	IV/SC	
Leuprolide	Lupron	90 min	50–80 20–30	SC IM depot	500–1000 µg/day 3.75–7.5 mg/month
Buserelin	Superfact, supercur	80 min	20–40	SC Intranasal	200–500 µg/day 300–400/3–4/day
Histrelin	Supprelin	<60 min	100	SC	100 µg/day
Goserelin	Zoladex	4.5 h	50–100	SC implant	3.6 mg/month
Nafarelin	Synarel	3–4 h	200	Intranasal	200–400/2/day
Triptorelin	Decapeptyl	3–4.2 h	36–144	SC IM depot	100-500 µg/day 3.75 mg/month

GONADOTROPIN RELEASING HORMONE ANTAGONIST[21,22]

Two different antagonist available are: (1) Cetrorelix and (2) Ganirelix.

It acts as a complete blocker for GnRH receptors and so blocks native GnRH that ultimately stops the release of FSH and LH from pituitary. It immediately blocks the gonadotropin release and the action is reversible. LH falls by 70% and FSH by 30% within 6 hours of antagonist administration.

Dosage of Antagonist

1. Daily dose scheme (day 1-5-6-7)
2. Single dose scheme (depot)

Daily dose scheme: In a daily dose scheme, 0.25 mg of cetrorelix or ganirelix is given daily.

Single dose scheme: In a single dose scheme, cetrorelix is given as 3 mg dose that inhibits LH surge for 4 days.

Both single and daily dose scheme gives an equivalent pregnancy rates.

Timings of antagonist: It can be given as fixed protocol or flexible protocol.[20,23,24]
- **Fixed protocol** is simpler and requires less monitoring. It should be started from day 5 of stimulation.
- **Flexible protocol** depends on endocrine and ultrasound criteria, which indicate the rise of LH.

Antagonist are given when the size of follicles is >-14 mm.

COMPARISON OF AGONISTS AND ANTAGONISTS[24-26]

GnRH agonist	GnRH antagonist
Downregulation of receptors	Inhibition of receptors without any activation
Desensitization of pituitary	Competitive antagonism
Flare-up response initially followed by downregulation	Immediate suppression
Slowly reversible response	Rapid reversible response
Longer IVF regimen	Shorter IVF regimen
Time consuming and more expensive	Less time and less expensive
More injections, inconvenient to the patient	Fewer injections increase patient compliance
No endogenous LH surge	Induction to endogenous LH

REFERENCES

1. Speroff L, Fritz MA. Clinical Gynecological Endocrinology and Infertility, 7th edition. Lippincott: Williams and Wilkins 2010.
2. Amer SAK. Polycystic ovarian syndrome: diagnosis and management of related infertility. Obstet Gynaecol Reprod Med. 2009;19(10):263-70.
3. ACOG. Infertility Workup for the Women's Health Specialist: ACOG Committee Opinion Summary, number 781. Obstet Gynecol. 2019; 133:1294-5.
4. Thessaloniki ESHRE/ASRM-Sponsored PCOS Consensus Workshop Group. Consensus on infertility Treatment Related to Polycystic Ovary Syndrome. Fertil Steril. 2008;89:505-22.
5. WHO-Scientific-Group. Agents stimulating gonadal function in the human. Report of a WHO Scientific Group. World Organ Tech Report Ser. 1973; 514:1-30.
6. Teede HJ, Misso ML, Costello MF, Dokras A, Laven J, Moran L, Piltonen T, Norman RJ; International PCOS Network. Recommendations from the International Evidence-based Guideline for the Assessment and Management of Polycystic Ovary Syndrome. Fertil Steril. 2018;110(3):364-79.
7. Smet ME, McLennan A. Rotterdam criteria, the end. Australas J Ultrasound Med. 2018;21(2):59-60. doi: 10.1002/ajum.12096. PMID: 34760503; PMCID: PMC8409808.
8. Gorlitsky GA, Kase NG, Speroff L. Ovulation and pregnancy rates with clomiphene citrate. Obstetrics and Gynecology 1978;51(3):265–9 [Internet]. [cited 2022 Nov 14].
9. Gysler M, March CM, Mishell DR, Bailey EJ. A decade's experience with an individualized clomiphene treatment regimen including its effect on the postcoital test. Fertil Steril. 1982;37(2):161-7 [Internet]. [cited 2022 Nov 14].
10. Morgante G, Massaro MG, di Sabatino A, Cappelli V, de Leo V. Therapeutic approach for metabolic disorders and infertility in women with PCOS. Gynecol Endocrinol. 2018;34(1):4-9.
11. Bordewijk EM, Ng KYB, Rakic L, Mol BWJ, Brown J, Crawford TJ, van Wely M. Laparoscopic ovarian drilling for ovulation induction in women with anovulatory polycystic ovary syndrome. Cochrane Database Syst Rev. 2020;2(2):CD001122. doi: 10.1002/14651858.CD001122.pub5. PMID: 32048270; PMCID: PMC7013239.
12. Nagori C, Panchal S. Handbook of Infertility and Ultrasound for Practicing Gynecologists. Google Books [Internet]. [cited 2022 Nov 14].
13. Bhatnagar AS. The discovery and mechanism of action of letrozole. Breast Cancer Research and Treatment [Internet]. [cited 2022 Nov 14] 2007;105(1):7–17.
14. Fouda UM, Sayed AM. Extended letrozole regimen versus clomiphene citrate for superovulation in patients with unexplained infertility undergoing intrauterine insemination: a randomized controlled trial. Reprod Biol Endocrinol. 2011;9:84. doi: 10.1186/1477-7827-9-84. PMID: 21693030; PMCID: PMC3135532.
15. Pritts EA. Letrozole for ovulation induction and controlled ovarian hyperstimulation. Curr Opin Obstet Gynecol. 2010;22(4):289-94.
16. Shi S, Hong T, Jiang F, Zhuang Y, Chen L, Huang X. Letrozole and human menopausal gonadotropin for ovulation induction in clomiphene resistance polycystic ovary syndrome patients: a randomized controlled study. Medicine (Baltimore). 2020;99(4):e18383. doi: 10.1097/MD.0000000000018383. PMID: 31977842; PMCID: PMC7004704.
17. Gardner DK, Weissman A, Howles CM, Shoham Z (Eds). Textbook of Assisted Reproductive Techniques, 4th edition, Volume 2: Clinical Perspectives. CRC Press. 2012, Jun 27.
18. Prapas Y, Ravanos K, Petousis S, Panagiotidis Y, Papatheodorou A, Margioula- Siarkou C, et al. GnRH antagonist administered twice the day before hCG trigger combined with a step-down protocol may prevent OHSS in IVF/ICSI antagonist cycles at risk for OHSS without affecting the reproductive outcomes: a prospective randomized control trial. Journal of Assisted Reproduction and Genetics. 2017;34(11):1537-45. [Internet]. [cited 2022 Nov 14]

19. Balasch J, Fábregues F, Creus M, Casamitjana R, Puerto B, Vanrell JA. Recombinant human follicle-stimulating hormone for ovulation induction in polycystic ovary syndrome: a prospective, randomized trial of two starting doses in a chronic low-dose step-up protocol. Journal of Assisted Reproduction and Genetics. 2000;17(10):561–5 [Internet]. [cited 2022 Nov 14].
20. Wang R, Lin S, Wang Y, Qian W, Zhou L. Comparisons of GnRH antagonist protocol versus GnRH agonist long protocol in patients with normal ovarian reserve: a systematic review and meta-analysis. PLoS One. 2017;12(4):e0175985 [Internet]. [cited 2022 Nov 14].
21. De Placido G, Mollo A, Clarizia R, Strina I, Conforti S, Alviggi C. Gonadotropin-releasing hormone (GnRH) antagonist plus recombinant luteinizing hormone vs. a standard GnRH agonist short protocol in patients at risk for poor ovarian response. Fertil Steril. 2006;85(1):247-50.
22. Borm G, Mannaerts B. Treatment with the gonadotropin-releasing hormone antagonist ganirelix in women undergoing ovarian stimulation with recombinant follicle stimulating hormone is effective, safe and convenient: results of a controlled, randomised, multicenter trial. The European Orgalutran Study Group. Hum Reprod. 2000; 15:1490-8.
23. Nelson SM, Yates RW, Lyall H, Jamieson M, Traynor I, Gaudoin M, et al. Anti-Müllerian hormone-based approach to controlled ovarian stimulation for assisted conception. Hum Reprod. 2009;24:867-77.
24. Ludwig M, Katalinic A, Banz C, Schroder AK, Loning M, Weiss JM, et al. Tailoring the GnRH antagonist cetrorelix acetate to individual patient's need in ovarian stimulation for IVF: results of a prospective, randomized study. Hum Reprod.2002;17(11):2842-5.
25. Griesinger G, Berndt H, Schultz L, Depenbusch M, Schultze-Mosgau A. Cumulative live birth rates after GnRH-agonist triggering of final oocyte maturation in patients at risk of OHSS: a prospective, clinical cohort study. Eur J Obstet Gynecol Reprod Biol. 2010; 149: 190–4
26. Bodri D, Sunkara SK, Coomarasamy A. Gonadotropin releasing hormone agonists versus antagonists for controlled ovarian hyperstimulation in oocyte donors: a systematic review and meta-analysis. Fertil Steril. 2011;95: 164–9

CHAPTER 9

Unexplained Infertility

Neharika Malhotra, Narendra Malhotra

■ INTRODUCTION

Infertility is when the couple fails to become pregnant in 12 months of unprotected intercourse in women <35 years of age and in 6-months for women >35 years of age.

Unexplained infertility (UI) is a diagnosis of exclusion when couple whose routine standard, basic investigations of infertility showed no abnormality and are unable to conceive within 1 year of trying, if under the age of 35 years and 6 months of trying, if over the age of 35 years.

Incidence for unexplained infertility is about 15–30%.[1]

Who should undergo infertility work-up?

- Women above 35 years of age should not wait and get evaluated as soon as possible and start treatment, if fail to conceive within 6 months.[2]
- Women above 40 years should receive expedited evaluation and treatment.[2]
- Women having any known conditions that can lead to infertility, such as irregular menstrual cycles and amenorrhea, suspected peritoneal disease or uterine causes, endometriosis, should also undertake immediate infertility work-up.[2]

Basic Infertility Work-up[2]	
Female	
History	Menstrual history, family history, current medications, presence of molimina (menstrual symptoms), coital frequency and timing, methods of contraception followed, any past surgery on the abdominal or pelvic region, use of nicotine, alcohol, or drug abuse, and any other serious illness
Physical	Examine all vital signs and include examination of thyroid, breast and pelvic region
Additional evaluation to identify the etiology of infertility	Evaluate ovarian reserve, ovulatory function and structural abnormalities using laboratory and imaging tests
Male	
History	Same as female history evaluation
Semen analysis	To evaluate semen volume, pH, sperm number, motility, agglutination and morphology

Unexplained infertility is a condition in which the basic infertility work-up fails to reveal any obvious abnormality. Patients with unexplained infertility should have evidence of ovulation by ultrasound, tubal patency checked by HSG or SSG and a normal semen analysis. Unexplained infertility was diagnosed in around 30% of infertile couples.[3]

Studies state that unexplained infertility represents the lower extreme of the normal distribution of fertility, or it can occur due to a defect in the fecundity which cannot be identified by basic infertility work-up. Also, diminished and delayed fecundity is found in couples with unexplained infertility.[3]

Since no correctable abnormality is observed in unexplained infertility, the therapy for unexplained infertility is empiric. Treatment regimens for managing unexplained infertility include intrauterine insemination (IUI), ovulation stimulation (OS) with oral or injectable medications, IUI with ovulation induction, and assisted reproductive technologies (ART).[3]

As we know that diagnosis of exclusion when couple whose routine standard, basic investigations of infertility showed no abnormality **(Flowchart 1)**:[1]

SOME PATHOLOGIES IDENTIFIED FOR UNEXPLAINED INFERTILITY

Some pathologies identified for unexplained infertility are illustrated in **Flowchart 2**.

FURTHER EVALUATION FOR UNEXPLAINED INFERTILITY

Female[4]

- *Laparoscopy:* Endometriosis, pelvic infections, altered pathology, adhesions
- *Hysteroscopy:* Endometritis, infections, tuberculosis, micropolyposis
- *Use of other procedures:* Contrast and methodized tests are not yet recommended, may have therapeutic role
- 3D Sonography
- *Test for tuberculosis*: HPE and culture are recommended. Evidence does not support—PCR
- Chlamydia
- *Endocrine and hormone evaluation:* Midluteal progesterone, TSH, PRL
- Genetic evaluation in selected cases.

Male[4]

- Varicocele
- Scrotal Doppler
- Endocrine evaluations
- Genetic evaluation in selected cases.

Basic Management (Flowchart 3)

- Proper evaluation of the couple
- Counseling regarding exercise and weight loss
- Counseling regarding avoidance of addictive habits (Smoking, tobacco and alcohol)

Flowchart 1: Diagnosis of UI.

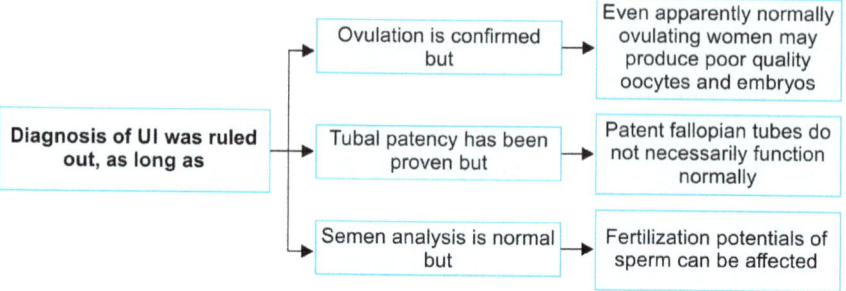

Flowchart 2: Unexplained infertility management protocol.

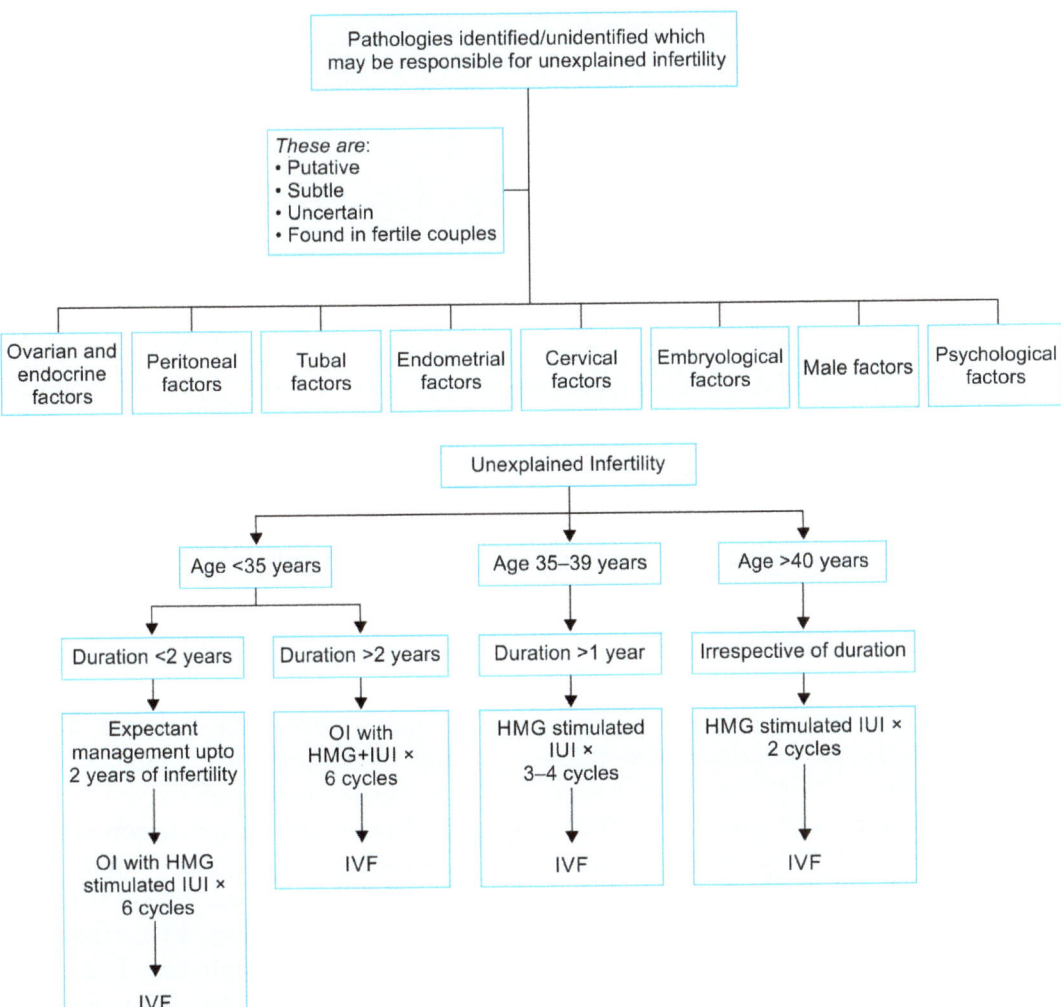

(HMG: human menopausal gonadotrophin; IUI: intrauterine insemination; OI: ovulation induction)

- Control of thyroid, diabetes and other endocrine issues
- *Treatment of infections:* Antibiotics coverage, if needed (Endometritis, tuberculosis and chlamydia)
- Probiotic supplementations
- Vitamin D supplementation
- Antioxidants where needed
- Correction of varicocele if needed.

EVIDENCE-BASED TREATMENTS FOR COUPLES WITH UNEXPLAINED INFERTILITY

A guideline by Practice Committee of the American Society for Reproductive Medicine 2019:

- There is good evidence that in couples who fail to achieve a pregnancy following a course of clomiphene citrate with IUI

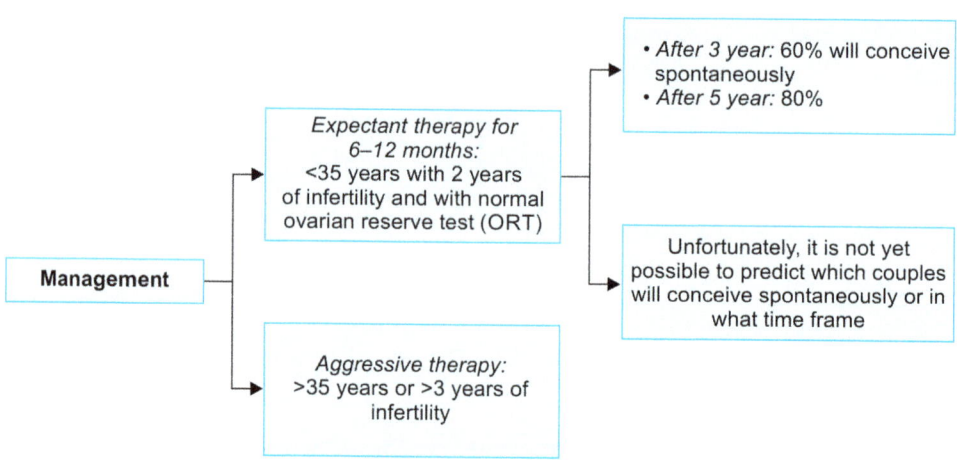

Flowchart 3: Basic management for UI.

treatment, immediate IVF results in a shorter time to pregnancy and lower cost per pregnancy than a strategy that incorporates gonadotropins with IUI treatments in women %40 years.
- There is good evidence that there is no reported difference in clinical pregnancy and live-birth rates when comparing IVF with conventional fertilization to IVF with ICSI in the setting of unexplained infertility. However, ICSI has been associated with higher fertilization rates and a reduced risk of complete fertilization failure as compared to conventional fertilization.
- It is recommended that couples with unexplained infertility initially undergo a course (typically 3 or 4 cycles) of OS and IUI with oral agents. For those unsuccessful with OS and IUI treatments with oral agents, IVF is recommended rather than OS and IUI with gonadotropins (Strength of Evidence: B; Strength of Recommendation: Moderate).

When to Do IVF/ICSI-ASRM 2019 Best Practice?

- As per ASRM guidelines, the current evidence does not support IVF as a first-line therapy over expectant management for 6 months in unexplained causes.[9]
- There is good evidence that immediate IVF in women at or above 38 years of age may be associated with a higher pregnancy rate and shorter time to pregnancy as compared to other treatment like OI/IUI or expectant management.
- It has been suggested that in couples who fail to achieve a pregnancy following a course of clomiphene citrate with IUI treatment, immediate IVF results in a shorter time to pregnancy and lower cost per pregnancy than IUI treatments in women of 40 years and this has been supported by good evidence.
- It has been reported no difference in clinical pregnancy and live-birth rates when comparing IVF with conventional fertilization to IVF with ICSI in the setting of unexplained infertility backed up by good evidence . However, ICSI has been associated with higher fertilization rates and a reduced risk of complete fertilization failure as compared to IVF.
- It is recommended that couples with unexplained infertility initially undergo

a course (typically 3 or 4 cycles) of OS and IUI with oral agents. For those unsuccessful with OS and IUI treatments with oral agents, IVF is recommended rather than OS and IUI with gonadotropins (Strength of Evidence: B; Strength of Recommendation: Moderate).

Luteal Support

- It has been studies about the benefit of luteal support in different cycles especially in gonadotropin cycles for OI-IUI.[9]
- While using clomiphene citrate, we must remember that initiates its ovulation-inducing effect at the level of the hypothalamus and therefore it competitively binds to estrogen receptors and preventing negative feedback of E2. Which increases GnRH pulse frequency, stimulating the release of LH and FSH from the anterior pituitary.[5] Increased LH may enhance corpus luteum function and increase both E2 and P in the luteal phase.[10]
- We also know that gonadotropins directly stimulate the ovaries to produce E2, which results in negative feedback at the levels of the hypothalamus and pituitary. The negative feedback disrupts the normal pulsatile release of LH and impairs P secretion from the corpus luteum. A shortened luteal phase has been demonstrated after OI with gonadotropins and has been associated with insufficient luteal phase serum P levels.
- Therefore, there is biologic plausibility for the benefit of exogenous P for luteal support in gonadotropin OI-IUI cycles.

RECOMMENDATIONS 2020 BY ASRM

- For unexplained infertility, it is not recommended directly to go for IUI as its not shown any benefit over expectant management (Strength of Evidence: A; Strength of Recommendation: Strong).
- ASRM does not recommend clomiphene with times intercourse as it has not shown any more benefit over expectant management (Strength of Evidence: B; Strength of Recommendation: Moderate).
- It is not recommended to use letrozole with timed intercourse as a treatment for unexplained infertility, as it is no more effective than expectant management (Strength of Evidence: B; Strength of Recommendation: Moderate).
- There has been no increase in pregnancy rate if gonadotropins are used with timed intercourse over expectant management (Strength of Evidence: B; Strength of Recommendation: Moderate)
- IUI with clomiphene citrate cycles is recommended for treatment for unexplained infertility (Strength of Evidence: A; Strength of Recommendation: Strong).
- ASRM recommends using letrozole with IUI to be considered as an alternative for couples with unexplained infertility, as studies to date suggest similar efficacy. Letrozole is considered an effective and well-tolerated option for ovulation induction (Strength of Evidence: A; Strength of Recommendation: Strong).
- It is not recommended to use letrozole or clomiphene citrate plus conventional-dose gonadotropins with IUI, as most studies associated with improved pregnancy rate over OS-IUI with oral medications are also associated with an increased risk of multiple-gestation pregnancy (Strength of Evidence: B; Strength of Recommendation: Moderate).
- ASRM does not recommend using gonadotropins with IUI as no studies have

shown an increase in the efficacy and this treatment becomes expensive and more complex (Moderate recommendation).
- Studies recommend single IUI options (Strength of Evidence: B; Strength of Recommendation: Moderate).
- It is recommended that couples with unexplained infertility can try 3-4 cycles of OI-IUI. For those unsuccessful with OI and IUI treatments with oral agents, IVF is recommended rather than OS and IUI with gonadotropins (Strength of Evidence: B; Strength of Recommendation: Moderate).

CONCLUSION

- The basic infertility work-up must be performed on any infertile patients.
- Older women (above 35 years) should receive expedited evaluation and undergo treatment.
- A complete medical history and proper family history must be obtained (both male and female partner).
- The examination of a female partner focuses on ovarian reserve, ovulatory function, and structural abnormalities.
- TVS must be done for all females to check the uterus, tubal patency and ovarian reserve.
- Low level of mid-luteal phase progesterone or short-luteal phase length was observed in patients after ovarian stimulation (a treatment for unexplained infertility).
- Also, treatment outcomes such as live birth rate were low when progesterone levels were low, proving that mid-luteal phase progesterone is a predictor of low odds of live birth and is associated with unexplained infertility treatment outcomes.
- Progesterone supplementation is mandatory during infertility treatment for excellent treatment outcomes (live birth and pregnancy rate).
- Progesterone supplementation should be initiated between oocyte retrieval and embryo transfer, with oocyte retrieval +1 day would be beneficial.[6]
- Co-administration of estrogen along with progesterone did not add any benefit to the treatment.[7]
- IM route of progesterone administration showed high clinical pregnancy rates.[7,8]
- Oral dydrogesterone is as effective as vaginal progesterone for LPS in women undergoing IUI, but serum progesterone levels and satisfaction rates in the dydrogesterone group were higher than the progesterone group.[6]

REFERENCES

1. Practice Committee of the American Society for Reproductive Medicine. Evidence-based treatments for couples with unexplained infertility: a guideline. Fertil Steril. 2020; 113(2):305-22.
2. Breitkopf DM. Infertility work-up for women's health specialist. ACOG Committee Opinion. Obstet Gynec.2019;133(6):e377-84.
3. Practice Committee of the American Society for Reproductive Medicine Effectiveness and treatment for unexplained infertility. Fertil Steril. 2006;86(5 Suppl 1):S111-4. doi: 10.1016/j.fertnstert.2006.07.1475.
4. Arpita R, Shah A, Gudi A, Homburg R. Unexplained infertility: an update and review of practice. Reproductive Bio Medicine Online. 2012;24:591-602.
5. Mohammed A, Woad KJ, Mann GE, et al. Evaluation of progestogen supplementation for luteal phase support in fresh in vitro fertilization cycles. Fertil Steril. 2019;112(3): 491-502.e3.
6. Zhang J, Du M, Li Z, Liu W, Ren B, Zhang Y, Guan Y. Comparison of dydrogesterone and medroxyprogesterone in the progestin-primed ovarian stimulation protocol for patients with poor ovarian response. Front

7. Labarta E, Mariani G, Holtmann N, et al. Low serum progesterone on the day of embryo transfer is associated with a diminished ongoing pregnancy rate in oocyte donation cycles after artificial endometrial preparation: a prospective study. Human Reproduction. 2017;32(12):2437-2.
8. Gaggiotti-Marre S, Martinez F, Coll L, Garcia S, Álvarez M, Parriego M, Barri PN, Polyzos N, Coroleu B. Low serum progesterone the day prior to frozen embryo transfer of euploid embryos is associated with significant reduction in live birth rates. Gynecol Endocrinol. 2019;35(5):439-42.
9. Chawla R, et al. A prospective study to correlate serum progesterone levels and clinical pregnancy outcome in frozen embryo transfer cycles. Fertil Sci Res. 2019;6(12):82-8.
10. Griesinger G, Blockeel C, Kahler E. Dydrogesterone as an oral alternative to vaginal progesterone for IVF luteal phase support: a systematic review and individual participant data meta-analysis. Main article. PLoS One. 2020;15(11):e0241044. doi: 10.1371/journal.pone.0241044.

Endocrinol (Lausanne). 2021;12:708704. doi: 10.3389/fendo.2021.708704. PMID: 34630325; PMCID: PMC8498200.

CHAPTER 10

Assisted Reproductive Techniques: When to Refer

Saeeda Wasim, Sharique Ahmad

■ INTRODUCTION

Assisted reproductive technology (ART) includes frozen embryo transfer, gamete intrafallopian transfer, zygote intrafallopian transfer, and IVF-ET (in vitro fertilization-embryo transfer). These methods also apply to gestational carriers and oocyte donation. IVF-ET is used in almost 99% of ART cycles. Many couples have had success conceiving thanks to IVF-ET. When previous therapies (such intrauterine insemination) have failed, ART may be referred.[1]

According to the American Center for Disease Control (CDC), ART are any fertility-related procedures that modify eggs or embryos. This concept excludes practices such as intrauterine inseminations where only sperm is altered. Procedures where ovarian stimulation is carried out without an intention for egg collection are also rejected from the concept of ovarian stimulation. IVF will be primarily examined, along with related procedures such as intracytoplasmic sperm injection and cryopreservation, since it is by far the most frequent ART therapy used (ICSI). ART are used to help people who are having trouble conceiving naturally achieve pregnancy.[2]

The information from further studies since the birth of Louise Brown, the first child born via in vitro fertilization, in the United Kingdom, there has been a persistently high rate of public interest in ART. Through the use of assisted reproductive technology pathological barriers including obstructed fallopian tubes and inoperable ovaries in females and a blocked oviducts and low levels of sperm in males can be avoided.[3]

Assistance with infertility is given through assisted reproduction. The term assisted a reproductive method refers to all fertility treatments that involve handling both the egg and the embryo. In these procedures, the woman's ovaries' eggs are surgically extracted, mixed in vitro with sperm, and the embryo is then placed back into the uterus. The most widely used assisted reproductive technology is in vitro fertilization (IVF). It starts with the removal of eggs from the ovary, is followed by in vitro fertilization, and is finished with the placement of the developing embryo in a uterus. Controlled ovarian stimulation, egg harvesting, fertilization, embryo culture, and embryo transfer are some of the steps that are involved. The procedure may also include intracytoplasmic sperm injection and preimplantation genetic testing. Then, extra embryos can be frozen or eggs or embryos can be preserved for fertility via cryopreservation with vitrification.[4]

■ TYPES OF ART

There are various ART approaches that use various methods and reproductive cells.

Depending on the situation, a specialist can suggest which ART is the most appropriate. In vitro fertilization is the most popular technique. IVF can be used to treat both unexplained infertility and infertility brought on by sperm antibodies, oligospermia, tubal dysfunction, or endometriosis. IVF completely omits the fallopian tubes for treating patients with tubal factor infertility.[5]

Other infertility causes treated with IVF include male factor infertility, reduced ovarian failure, ovarian reserve, unexplained infertility and ovulatory dysfunction.[6] IVF can be done with a gestational carrier in individuals for whom pregnancy is often contraindicated (described below) or who have uterine factor infertility. Outside of infertile conditions, IVF is also employed. Those who want preimplantation genetic testing prior to conception (such as those who are known to be carriers of specific genetic abnormalities), fertility preservation (such as before gonadotoxic therapy), or patients who want to put off having children can utilize it. If these ladies are in a committed relationship, they may choose to preserve their eggs or embryos.[7]

PGT testing may involve preimplantation genetic diagnosis to look for specific dangerous inherited illnesses or preimplantation genetic screening (PGS) to rule out aneuploidy.

Gamete Intrafallopian Tube Transfer (GIFT)

Since IVF has a higher success rate than GIFT, then GIFT is a less common alternative. When a woman has unexplained infertility, normal tubal function, and endometriosis, GIFT is most frequently employed. In GIFT, the gametes are first collected in a tube of eggs and sperm before being surgically inserted into the fallopian tubes. A person does not have to select which embryo to transfer because there is no IVF procedure.

Intracytoplasmic Sperm Injection (ICSI)

When other strategies are failing or are likely to fail, this one can be helpful. The number of sperm cells in the ejaculate is too low for IVF, there is a significant sperm abnormality present, and fertilization failed after receiving standard IVF treatment. ICSI is the term used to describe the procedure in which one sperm is manually inserted into an egg for fertilization while being seen by extremely powerful microscopes. IVF is different from ICSI in that several sperm and eggs are combined inside of a tube during IVF. The embryologists watch as the sperm and egg naturally combine. ICSI is helpful when using sperm from the testicles or in cases of severe male infertility.

Zygote Intrafallopian Transfer (ZIFT)

IVF and GIFT are combined to create ZIFT. Before placing fertilized eggs or zygotes back into the fallopian tubes, specialists use IVF techniques to stimulate and collect the eggs. ZIFT has the potential to assist those who have seriously affected fallopian tubes or infertility concerns conceive.[8] After IVF, a technique known as zygote Intrafallopian transfer involves moving the fertilized egg's zygote (which has not yet split) into the oviduct.[9]

Pronuclear Stage Tubal Transfer (PROST)

Similar to ZIFT, pronuclear stage tubal transfer (PROST) involves moving a fertilized egg to the reproductive tract before cell division has place.[8]

Controlled ovarian stimulation, in which women get hormone therapy to stimulate the release of additional eggs from the ovaries.

Egg donation, in which a recipient receives donated eggs from a third party donor so they can use assisted reproductive technologies to become pregnant.

Egg freezing is a method through which a woman who wants to maintain her fertility might store her eggs for future use.

Sperm freezing is a procedure where the sperm is preserved to protect the man's fertility, either before undergoing a medical procedure that can affect fertility or to be utilized as donor sperm in the future.

In a testicular biopsy, a small sample of tissue is taken from the scrotum after a cut is formed around it. To identify the underlying cause of male infertility, a biopsy is performed.

The procedure known as testicular sperm aspiration (TESA) is used to remove tissue or sperm from a man's testis. It is typical to collect the sperm on the same day as the female partners' eggs for IVF or IUI cycles.

Therapeutic donor insemination (TDI), in which sperm from a recognized or unidentified donor is injected into the uterus around the ovulation time. Before the procedure, the sperm may have been frozen and thawed.

Another method that enjoys about the same level of popularity as IVF is intrauterine insemination (IUI). The procedure is known as "insemination," and it differs from IVF in that the sperm is inserted into the woman's womb at the moment of ovulation. Embryo freezing is a procedure that allows you to freeze an embryo for use in IVF later on.

A woman who has failed to become pregnant after three straight IVF cycles can undergo ERA testing to determine the causes of implantation failure.[10]

CLINICAL CONDITION TO REFER FOR ART (MALE AND FEMALE FACTOR INFERTILITY)

The issue of infertility is getting worse today, not just in western countries but also in other regions as even in developing nations, couples postpone having children until they are well past the age of 30, preferring to concentrate on their careers and financial security.[11] Additionally, there are some diseases that can cause infertility. Many infertile patients who desire children have sought treatment with assisted reproductive technology and may benefit from it (ART) because its success rates are anticipated to be higher than those of current treatments. ART is utilized for all types of infertility issues. The second most common reason for using assisted reproductive technology is infertility.[12]

Male and female factor infertility like:

Unexplained Infertility

Those who have an isolated defect in one partner, those who have several problems in one or both partners, and those who are infertile without obvious cause (no apparent defect in either partner. When testing shows no evident reason for your fertility issues, doctors refer to infertility as "unexplained infertility." Only when both partners have undergone thorough fertility assessments do providers make the diagnosis of unexplained infertility. These tests frequently show:
- No structural problems with your uterus or uterine anomalies
- Regular interval ovulation

- Your fallopian tubes are unobstructed and open.
- Your egg count is healthy (ovarian reserve).
- The hormones required for reproduction are produced in your brain in regular amounts.
- The results of your partner's semen analysis are normal (count, amount, motility and shape).

Female Factor Infertility

When tubal and peritoneal disease cannot be treated with microsurgical methods and the patient also has tuberculosis, bilateral hydrosalpinx, and inaccessible ovaries, this condition is known as tubal disease. An obstruction in the fallopian tubes prevents the egg and sperm from contacting one other, resulting in tubal factor infertility. 25–30% of all cases of infertility are caused by the tubal factor. The syndrome can cause one or more fallopian tubes to be fully closed, only have one blocked tube, or have scarring constrict the tubes.[13]

Women with severe intrauterine adhesions who are resistant to surgical rupture of the adhesion and patients who have had their ovaries removed can transfer their embryos to surrogates through IVF. Other uterine variables include Müllerian agenesis and congenital uterine defects.

Absolute uterine factor is one of the female causes of infertility. A lady with infertility is unable to conceive when her uterus is absent or fully non-functional.

Included in this category are infertility issues brought on by polyps, scar tissue, fibroids, radiation damage, or uterine injuries that hinder conception. In the rare illness known as Asherman syndrome, the uterus' scar tissue forms adhesions, which act as physical barriers inside the uterus and hinder pregnancy.[14]

Ovarian-related problems in women oligo-ovulation, hypogonadotropic anovulation, and severe polycystic ovarian syndrome (PCOS). Approximately 15% of infertile couples and 40% of infertile women have ovulatory abnormalities. Three menstrual irregularities are frequently the result of a deficiency in ovulatory function, which is typically detectable by history in the majority of women. Menstrual irregularities should be looked into in patients to rule out underlying conditions such polycystic ovarian syndrome, thyroid issues, hyperprolactinemia, and hypothalamic reasons related to weight changes. Eumenorrhea, normal menstrual cycles based on history is a highly accurate indicator of ovulation, and only a very tiny percentage of eumenorrheic patients have anovulatory serum progesterone levels (3 ng/mL).[15]

There is an imbalance in the female sex hormones in women who have PCOS, also known as polycystic ovarian syndrome. The imbalance can stop mature eggs from developing and releasing. Neither ovulation nor pregnancy can take place in the absence of a developed egg. An abnormal rise in the hormone testosterone, which is largely a male sex hormone, may also be a sign of hormonal imbalance. Testosterone is also produced by women, Albeit often in much lower concentrations.

Insulin resistance is common in PCOS-afflicted women. The body's failure to properly reduce blood sugar levels is known as insulin resistance. Too much insulin is produced when blood sugar levels are too high. The synthesis of testosterone is also increased by excess insulin, which contributes to several PCOS symptoms.[16]

Endometriosis: Endometriosis in women who have undergone unsuccessful medicinal or surgical treatment and is moderate to severe. In the overall female population, endometriosis affects 6–10% of women, and it affects 35–50% of women who have pain, infertility, or both. Endometriosis is 6–8 times more common in infertile women than in fertile ones. There is still no consensus regarding the cause of the relation between endometriosis and infertility, despite substantial research, and a number of possible explanations have been put forth. These pathways include distorted pelvic structure, endocrine and ovarian disorders, changed peritoneal function, and changed endometrial hormonal and cell-mediated functions. Women who have experienced early menopause, genetic disorders, or radiation therapy may also be referred for care and ART.[17]

Male Factor Infertility

Semen abnormalities in men include oligozoospermia, low sperm counts, and non-obstructive and obstructive azoospermia and. A male's inability to cause pregnancy in a fertile female is known as male infertility. A change in sperm concentration, motility, or morphology is considered a sign of male factor infertility in at least one samples of two sperm analyses taken 1 and 4 weeks apart. It affects about 7% of all men in humans and causes 40–50% of infertility. Semen quality is utilized as a proxy for an assessment of male fecundity since male infertility is sometimes caused by inadequacies in the semen.[18]

ESHRE GUIDELINES FOR REFERRAL

ESHRE advises ART centers to implement this guidance after first adhering to local and/or national laws and recommendations from local and/or national governments on COVID-19.

a. High-risk patients should wait to begin ART treatment until it has been pronounced safe to do so by appropriate medical specialists and/or local health authorities (e.g., those with diabetes, hypertension, using immunosuppressive medicine, previous transplant patients, lung, liver, or renal disease).
b. All patients should be given the option of starting or delaying their ART treatment. Patient preferences should be carefully recorded in both situations.
c. Patients must receive thorough information, comprehend the hazards of COVID-19 disease, and realize that these risks are enhanced in cases of infection during pregnancy. Also, patients must be instructed on ways to lower their risk of infection generally.
d. The Code of Conduct must be signed by all patients and followed.[19]

ASRM GUIDELINES FOR REFERRAL

The ASRM meeting provided evidence that the addition of insurance coverage for infertility therapies could enhance the present oversight of ART. Such protection could encourage the use of the most medically necessary techniques and lower the incidence of multiple births, along with the costs and hazards that come with them. By mandating adherence to ASRM guidelines or the performance of ART procedures only at clinics subject to SART standards, insurance coverage for infertility might also improve current monitoring and quality controls.[20]

The ASRM and SART recommendations for informed consent should be followed by assisted reproductive technology procedures. SART has created consent forms that its members are free to use or modify for their particular medical setting. Prior to performing any procedure, the laboratory needs proof of informed consent permission.[21]

The American Society for Reproductive Medicine's (ASRM) Practice Committee has developed recommendations for a typical infertility assessment. Included are hysterosalpingogram, ovulation assessment and semen analysis, screening for ovarian reserve, and, if required, laparoscopy. When the results of a conventional infertility evaluation are normal, the diagnosis of unexplained infertility is made. Though estimates vary, there is a 15–30% chance that all test results for an infertile couple are normal and unrelated. It is important to keep in mind that patient characteristics differ between programs, thus comparisons between treatment facilities should not be made using success rates.[22]

Each patient is assessed prior to beginning ART to increase her chances of success and a healthy pregnancy. Before trying conception, chronic medical disorders such as diabetes, hypertension, and asthma should be under good control.

If immunity is low, then vaccination can be given prior to conception. People who run a high risk of passing down particular genetic illnesses to their offspring can be advised about the inheritance and progression of the condition and referred for potential therapies such preimplantation genetic testing.

Women's capacity to conceive declines with age, and their risk of miscarriage increases the amount of oocytes that are currently potentially available for fertilizations is known as the ovarian reserve and can be measured using serum testing or ultrasounds.

Tests for ovarian reserve are reliable indicators of how the body may react to ovarian stimulation. Tests for anti-Müllerian hormone (AMH), FSH levels, and estradiol, antral follicle count as determined by ultrasound. Usually, an uterine evaluation occurs before an IVF.

Review of a semen analysis is necessary. Over time, sperm quality changes could take place and have an impact on IVF outcomes.[23]

■ ADVANTAGES OF ART

- ART describes medical techniques intended to achieve pregnancy. Many patients who might not otherwise be able to become pregnant benefit from ART. Having a successful pregnancy and a healthy baby is ART's main benefit. IVF can help people who otherwise would not be able to have children achieve this.
- The best chance for women who have blocked or damaged fallopian tubes to conceive a child using their own eggs is through ART (IVF).
- IVF can be used to increase the likelihood that older patients can conceive in cases where they are older or have a poor ovarian reserve.
- *Unexplained infertility:* 1 in 6 couples will experience fertility issues, and sometimes these can go misdiagnosed even after examination. An intervention may be beneficial for these patients.
- *PCOS:* IVF has been quite effective for PCOS patients who have trouble becoming pregnant naturally or with ovulation induction.
- *Endometriosis:* Patients with endometriosis, in which portions of the womb-lining grow outside the womb, may choose to undergo IVF because it has been successful in this population.
- *Premature ovarian failure:* IVF using donor eggs, which normally has high success rates.

- It is possible to check embryos for inherited illnesses. IVF with pre-implantation genetic diagnosis (PGD) is one of the most reliable techniques for people who are known carriers of genetic conditions including cystic fibrosis, Huntington's disease, and muscular dystrophy to guarantee that a child conceived will not be affected by the condition.
- Pre-implantation genetic screening (PGS), which checks embryos for chromosomal abnormalities including Down's syndrome, can increase the likelihood of a favorable outcome.[24]

DISADVANTAGES OF ART

Even though assisted reproductive technologies (ARTs) are common practices used globally, there are still lots of safety-related problems that need to be resolved. Infertility and ART may be linked to hazards that are inherent to conception, delivery, and infancy, infertility itself and its causes, and risks that are iatrogenic to ART. Although there are several possible hazards connected to ART, it is now obvious that multiple pregnancy and its effects provide the most threat. Although significant efforts should be made to lower the danger of multiple gestations during IVF, it is equally obvious that single-embryo transfers are not always the best option.[25, 26]

Another study reveals at this point, there are still worries about the effects of irregularities in genomic imprinting, as well as dangers related to culture conditions and even our environment. Only time will tell if children born after ART are more likely to grow up with specific chronic illnesses than other children. In any scenario, the risks to mothers and babies born through IVF are likely to remain higher than those for moms and babies born naturally and without medical intervention.

The vast majority of pregnancies and children have been essentially "normal" and there have been over 5 million births following ART worldwide, so it is clear that any increased risk must be minimal.[27]

REFERENCES

1. Park K, Allard-Phillips E, Christman G, Dimza M, Rhoton-Vlasak A. Assisted reproductive technologies and their association with adverse pregnancy outcomes and long-term cardiovascular disease: implications for counseling patients. Current Treatment Options in Cardiovascular Medicine. 2021;23(8):1-1.
2. Jain M, Singh M. Assisted Reproductive Technology (ART) Techniques. InStatPearls [Internet] 2021 Dec 4. StatPearls Publishing.
3. Kamel RM. Assisted reproductive technology after the birth of Louise Brown. Journal of Reproduction and Infertility. 2013;14(3):96-109.
4. Amjad S, Rehman R. Assisted reproductive techniques. InSubfertility 2021 Jan 1 (pp. 185-197). Elsevier.
5. Reddy UM, Wapner RJ, Rebar RW, Tasca RJ. Infertility, assisted reproductive technology, and adverse pregnancy outcomes: executive summary of a National Institute of Child Health and Human Development workshop. Obstetrics and Gynecology. 2007;109(4):967-77.
6. https://www.msdmanuals.com/en-in/professional/gynecology-and-obstetrics/infertility/assisted-reproductive (Internet)
7. van Eekelen R, van Geloven N, van Wely M, Bhattacharya S, van der Veen F, Eijkemans MJ, McLernon DJ. IVF for unexplained subfertility; whom should we treat? Hum Reprod. 2019;34(7):1249-59. [PMC free article] [PubMed]
8. Noyes N, Labella PA, Grifo J, Knopman JM. Oocyte cryopreservation: a feasible fertility preservation option for reproductive age cancer survivors. J Assist Reprod Genet. 2010;27(8):495-9. [PMC free article] [PubMed]
9. Reproductive Ethics: New Reproductive Technologies. Rachel A Ankeny, in

International Encyclopedia of Public Health (Second Edition), (Internet) 2017.
10. https://www.sitarambhartia.org/blog/gynecology/infertility/assisted-reproductive-technology/ (Internet).
11. Quaas A, Dokras A. Diagnosis and treatment of unexplained infertility. Reviews in Obstetrics and Gynecology. 2008;1(2):69.
12. Klitzman R. Gatekeepers for infertility treatment? Views of ART providers concerning referrals by non-ART providers. Reproductive Biomedicine and Society Online. 2018;5:17-30.
13. https://www.columbiadoctors.org/treatments-conditions/tubal-factor-infertility-fallopian-tube-obstruction).
14. https://my.clevelandclinic.org/health/diseases/17738-uterine-factor (Internet).
15. Zhao L, Zhu Z, Lou H, Zhu G, Huang W, Zhang S, Liu F. Polycystic ovary syndrome (PCOS) and the risk of coronary heart disease (CHD): a meta-analysis. Oncotarget. 2016;7(23):33715.
16. https://www.medicalnewstoday.com/articles/312841 (Internet).
17. Bulletti C, Coccia ME, Battistoni S, Borini A. Endometriosis and Infertility. Journal of Assisted Reproduction and Genetics. 2010;27(8):441-7.
18. Kumar N, Singh AK. Trends of male factor infertility: an important cause of infertility: a review of literature. Journal of Human Reproductive Sciences. 2015;8(4):191.
19. Vermeulen N, Ata B, Gianaroli L, Lundin K, Mocanu E, Rautakallio-Hokkanen S, Tapanainen JS, Veiga A. A picture of medically assisted reproduction activities during the COVID-19 pandemic in Europe. Human Reproduction Open. 2020;2020(3):hoaa035.
20. Practice Committees of the American Society for Reproductive Medicine and Society for Assisted Reproductive Technology. Recommendations for practices utilizing gestational carriers: an ASRM Practice Committee Guideline. Fertil Steril. 2017; 107:e3-10.
21. Society for Assisted Reproductive Technology. Member resources: consent forms. Available at: https://www.sart.org/professionals-and-providers/sartmembers/.
22. Mastenbroek S, de Wert G, Adashi EY. The imperative of responsible innovation in reproductive medicine. New England Journal of Medicine. 2021;385(22):2096-100.
23. https://www.sart.org/patients/sart-patient-evaluation/.
24. https://www.createfertility.co.uk/blog/the-advantages-and-disadvantages-of-ivf.
25. Rebar RW. What are the risks of the assisted reproductive technologies (ART) and how can they be minimized? Reproductive Medicine and Biology. 2013;12(4):151-8.
26. Jones Jr HW. The use of controlled ovarian hyperstimulation (COH) in clinical in vitro fertilization: the role of Georgeanna Seegar Jones. Fertil Steril. 2008;90(5):e1-3.
27. Källén B, Finnström O, Lindam A, Nilsson E, Nygren KG, Olausson PO. Cancer risk in children and young adults conceived by in vitro fertilization. Pediatrics. 2010;126(2):270-6.

Index

Page numbers followed by *f* refer to figure, *fc* refer to flowchart, and *t* refer to table.

A

Acne 53
Adenomyosis 8, 37
Adhesions 38
Adipose tissue 26
Adnexa 38, 42*f*
Adrenal hyperplasia,
    congenital 53
Androgen deficiency 3
Androgens 26
Anorexia 26
Anovulation 53
  causes of 52
Antagonist 54, 58
  dosage of 58
  timings of 58
Anti-Müllerian hormone 6
  tests for 73
Antioxidants 20, 28
Antral follicular count 6, 39
Applebaum score 8
Aromatase inhibitors 55
Artificial reproductive
    techniques 44, 70
  advancement of 1, 73
  disadvantages of 74
  types of 68
Ascorbic acid effects 28
Asherman syndrome 71
Aspirin, low-dose 55
Assisted reproductive technology 25, 57, 68, 74
Asthenozoospermia 4, 13
Azoospermia 12, 22
  non-obstructive 13
  obstructive 13
Azoospermic genes 13

B

Basic infertility 66
  work-up 61
Beads-on-a-string 41
Bisphenol acetate 17
Blocked tube 71
Body mass index 53
Bulimia nervosa 26

C

Carbohydrates 27
Celiac disease 25
Cervix 5
Chlamydia trachomatis 46
Clomiphene 55
  citrate 54, 55, 65
  dose of 54
Cogwheel sign 41, 41*f*
Coital disorder 10
Color Doppler 8
Contraception 10
Controlled ovarian stimulation 70
Corpus luteum 39
Cul-de-sac tenderness 5
Cycle, monitoring of 42
Cyst 39
  follicular 39

D

Deoxyribonucleic acid repair
    genes 24
Dermoid cyst 40
  bilateral 40*f*
Diabetes 12
Diethylstilbestrol 11
Digital rectal examination 12
Distal tubal disease 50
Dyspareunia 2

E

Echogenicity, cyst with
    internal 39
Egg
  donation 70
  freezing 70
Ejaculatory duct 3
Embryo 68
  culture 68
  development 22
  freezing 70
  transfer 44, 68
Embryogenesis 16
Endocrinal disorders 12
Endocrine 62
  disrupting chemical 16, 18*f*
  effects 17, 18*f*
  factor 7
Endocrinopathy 12
Endometrial
  cyst 40*f*
  pattern 37
  polyp 38, 38*f*
  sampling 7
  thickness 37, 43
  vascularity 43
Endometrioma 40
Endometriosis 22, 72, 73
Endometritis 38
Endometrium 37, 37*f*
Environmental protection
    agency 16
Epididymides 12
Estradiol, endogenous 28

F

Fallopian tube 46
  dilated 48
  effect on 17
  normal 47*f*
  ultrasound evaluation of 47
Falloposcopy 6, 48
Fatty acid
  dietary 27
  polyunsaturated 27
Fertility 46
  diet 25
  external agents on 20*f*
Fertilization 16, 68
Fetuses, female 23
Fibroid 35
  classification of 36*f*
Folates 28
Folic acid 20
  supplements 28

Index

Follicle, assessment of 42
Follicle-stimulating
    hormone 4, 23
    preparations 56
Follicular monitoring 6
Folliculogenesis, defects in 24

G

Gamete intrafallopian tube
    transfer 69
Gametogenesis 16
Genetic 22, 23
    abnormality 53
        specific 69
    diagnosis, pre-implantation 74
    polymorphisms 22
    testing, preimplantation 69
Germline mosaicism 23
Gonadotoxins 11
Gonadotropin 55
    releasing hormone 53, 55
        agonist 57
        antagonist 58
    therapy, different regimens
        of 56

H

Hirsutism 53
Homocysteine, lower 28
Hormonal tests 5
Hormone 17
    evaluation 62
Human fertility, effects on 21
Human infertility genes 24
Human menopausal
        gonadotropin 56, 63
Hydrosalpinx 42*f*
    S-shaped 41*f*
Hypergonadotropic
        hypogonadism 52, 53
Hyperinsulinemia 7
    lowering 27
Hyperprolactinemia 53, 71
Hyperspermia 3
Hypertension 12
Hypogonadotropic
        hypogonadism 10, 52
Hypothalamic-pituitary
    gonadal axis 17
    ovarian axis 52
Hypothalamus, effect on 17
Hysterosalpingogram 4

Hysterosalpingography 46
    complications of 47
    contrast 48
Hysteroscopy 48, 62

I

In vitro fertilization 68
    advantages of 49
    disadvantages of 49
Infections, treatment of 63
Infertile couples 2
    evaluation of 1
Infertility 1, 22, 25, 52, 72
    anovulatory 52
    basic evaluation 1*f*
    causes of 10
    conventional 73
    correlates, frequency of 25
    environment and 16
    evaluation 2, 11
    female 22, 23, 25, 70, 71
        causes of 71
    male 10, 14, 22, 70, 72
    primary male 10
    start work-up for 2
    treatment of 8
    types of 27
    ultrasound evaluation of 33
    work-up 61
Inflammation 3
Insulin 7, 26
    resistance 71
    sensitizing agents 55
Intracytoplasmic sperm
        injection 27, 69
Intramural fibroid 36
Intrauterine insemination 62, 63,
    68, 70

K

Klinefelter syndrome 13

L

Laparoscopy 48, 62
Lesions
    complex 40
    solid 40
Letrozole 55, 65
    step-up protocol 55
    therapy, extended 55
Lipids 27

Liquefaction 3
Luteal progesterone 7
Luteinizing hormone 4, 12, 23, 52

M

Malnutrition 26
Mature follicle 42
    characteristics of 42
Mediterranean diet 29
    patterns 25
Meigs' syndrome 40
Menstrual irregularities 71
Metformin 55
Microbiota composition 25
Microdose flare protocol 57
Minerals 28
Mitochondrial dysfunction 24
Monosomy X 23
Motile cells, percentage of 4
Motility 72
    type of 4
Mycobacterium tuberculosis 46
Myoma 8
Myometrium 35, 37*f*
    anterior 37*f*

N

Neisseria gonorrhoeae 46
Nipple discharge 5
Non-steroidal anti-inflammatory
    drugs 46
Normogonadotropic
        normogonadism 52, 53
Nutrition 25
    healthy 26

O

Obesity 53
Oligospermia 12
    severe 13
Oligozoospermia 12, 22
Omega-3 fatty acids 27
Oocyte
    retrieved, number of 17
    survival 17
Oogenesis 23
    defects in 22
Oral dydrogesterone 66
Ovarian factor 6
Ovarian failure 53, 69
    premature 23, 53, 73

Index

Ovarian reserve 69, 71
   tests for 73
Ovarian stimulation 68
Ovarian torsion 40
Ovary 17
   evaluation of 33, 39
   lesions of 39
Ovulation
   healthy 26
   induction 63
      medical options for 54
   predictor kits 7
   signs of 42
   stimulation 62
Ovulatory disorder 53
Ovulatory dysfunction 69

P

Pelvic
   disorders 6
   inflammatory disease 46
Peritubal adhesions 47
Phallus 12
Polychlorinated biphenyls 16
Polycystic ovarian
   disease 39, 39f
   syndrome 22, 23, 53, 71, 73
Polyp 8
Progesterone supplementation 66
Pronuclear stage tubal transfer 69
Prostatic lytic enzymes, lack of 3
Protein 26, 27
Pulsatility index 8
Pyospermia 14

R

Reproductive
   capacity 17
   cells 68
   efficiency 27
   health 16
   tract
      development 22
      infections 2
Resistivity index 42

S

Saline infusion 8
Salpingitis isthmic nodosa 47
Salpingoscopy 6, 48
Scrotum 12

Semen
   analysis 3, 12
   microscopy of 4
   parameters 11t
      normal 3, 22
   report 5
Seminal plasma
         microenvironment,
         effects 17
Septation, incomplete 41f
Serum progesterone 6, 54
Sex hormone-binding globulin
   7, 28
Sexually transmitted infections 2
Sonohysterogram 4
Sonosalpingography 6
Spasm 47
Sperm
   cells 69
   concentration 4, 72
   count 4
      decreased 12
      total 4
   freezing 70
   function tests 5
   in ejaculate, absence of 12
   low levels of 68
   morphology 5
   motility 4
      decreased 13
   viability 4, 13
Spermatozoa 5
Steroid hormones 17
Stress, psychological 13
String sign, beads on 41
Subfertility, translation of 21
Submucosal fibroid 36f
Subserosal fibroid 36
Synechiae 38, 39f

T

Testes 12
Testicular
   atrophy 14
   biopsy 5, 70
   disorders 11
   injury 11
   sperm aspiration 70
Testosterone 12
Therapeutic donor
         insemination 70
Thyroid
   disorders 53
   issues 71

Transrectal ultrasonography 14
Transvaginal sonography 33
Trophoblastic steroidogenesis 28
Truncal obesity 12
Tubal disease 71
Tubal factor 6
   infertility 46
   management of 46
Tubal infertility, evaluation of 46
Tubal inflammation 42
Tubal inflammatory disease 46
Tubal lesions 41
Tubal ligation reversal 49
Tubal pathologies 49
Tubal polyps 47
Tubal surgery
   advantages of 49
   disadvantages of 49
Tube, evaluation of 33
Tuberculosis
   test for 62
   tubal 47
Tuboplasty 49
Turner's syndrome 23

U

Ultrashort protocol 57
Ultrasonography 44
   guided oocyte 44
Ultrasound 33
Unexplained infertility 5, 61-63,
        69, 70, 73
   basic management for 64fc
   diagnosis of 62fc
   evaluation for 62
   management protocol 63fc
Urine analysis 5
   postejaculatory 14
Uterine
   anomaly, classification of 34t,
      35t
   biophysical score 43
   blood flow 43
   corpus 5
   factor 5
      absolute 71
      infertility 69
   fibroids 22
Uterus 33f
   animal, effects on 17
   arcuate 34f
   bicornuate 33f, 34f
   evaluation of 33

normal 33*f*
septate 33*f*, 34*f*
subseptate 33*f*
unicornuate 33*f*, 34

V

Vaginismus 2
Varicocele 14
Vas deferens 12
    absence of 14
Vitamin 28
    C 30

W

Waist sign 41, 41*f*
Weight disorders
    female 19
    male 19

X

X-chromosome 23
    abnormalities 24
    inactivation 29
XX gonadal dysgenesis 24

Y

Y-chromosome
    microdeletions 13
    screening for 22
Y-microdeletion studies 13

Z

Zygote intrafallopian transfer 69

EU GSPR Authorised Reprsentative
Logos Europe, 9 rue Nicolas Poussin
1700, La Rochelle, France
Phone: +33 (0) 6 67 93 73 78
E-mail: contact@logoseurope.eu

www.ingramcontent.com/pod-product-compliance
Ingram Content Group UK Ltd.
Pitfield, Milton Keynes, MK11 3LW, UK
UKHW050132170426
5217IPUK00053BA/1297